Duke & the Doctor

HEALTH BEGINS IN THE COLON

Dr. Edward F. Group III, DC, ND, DACBN

SENIOR EDITOR
Dr. Edward F. Group III, DC, ND, DACBN

ASSISTANT EDITOR
David Tubbs

BOOK LAYOUT AND DESIGN
Nida Ali

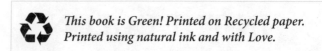 *This book is Green! Printed on Recycled paper. Printed using natural ink and with Love.*

NOTE: The statements made in this book have not been evaluated by the FDA and are not intended to diagnose, treat, cure or prevent any disease. **Health Begins in the Colon** and related media are provided for informational purposes only.

Health Begins in the Colon
Copyright © 2007 by Dr. Edward F. Group III
All rights reserved.

This edition published by Global Healing Center, Inc.
For information, address:

2040 North Loop West
Suite 108
Houston, TX 77018
www.ghchealth.com

Published in the United States of America. No part of this book may be used or reproduced in any manner without the written permission of the publisher.
ISBN 10: 0-9801449-0-6
ISBN 13: 978-0-9801449-0-1

Table of Contents

PART ONE:
How Disease Starts and Health Begins in the Colon

CHAPTER 1
The Secret to Health
1

- 2 So What Is the Secret to Health?
- 4 Why Has This Been Kept a "Secret"?
- 6 What Happens When You Have a Toxic Intestine, Colon, or Liver?

CHAPTER 2
What is a Toxic Colon?
13

- 16 What Exactly Does the Colon Do?
- 17 What Causes the Colon to Malfunction in the First Place?
- 18 How Clogged Are Our Colons?
- 22 Examples of Potential Daily Toxin Intake

CHAPTER 3
Conditions of a Toxic Colon
27

- 29 Constipation: What Is It?
- 31 IBS: What Is Irritable Bowel Syndrome?
- 34 Diverticular Disease: What Is It?
- 37 Celiac Disease: What Is It?
- 39 Inflammatory Bowel Disease: What Is It?
- 43 Colon Polyps: What Are They?
- 44 Colon Cancer: What Is It?

CHAPTER 4
How Healthy is Your Colon?
49

    50 The Bristol Stool Scale
    52 Analyzing Your Stool
    54 How Do I Identify Mucous in My Stool?
    55 What Do Colored Stools Indicate?
    58 Take the Colon Health Self-Test

CHAPTER 5
The Oxygen Colon Cleanse
61

    70 Benefits of Oxygen in the Body
    76 The 6-Day Oxygen Colon Cleanse
    78 6 TIPS to Maximize the Oxygen Colon Cleanse
    87 Questions & Answers on the 6-Day Oxygen Colon Cleanse
    90 The Overnight "Quick Colon Cleanse"
    91 Can I Use Any Other Colon Cleansing Methods?
    94 Which Herbal Colon Cleansing Ingredients Should Concern Me?
   104 Can I Do Anything Else To Help Keep My Colon Healthy?

CHAPTER 6
The Colon Diet
111

   112 The Human Body's Biorhythms
   113 What is the Best Diet Plan for the Health of My Colon?
   119 General Recommended Diet Plan

PART TWO:

How to Live in a Green, Toxin-Free Environment

CHAPTER 7
How to Reduce Intestinal Toxins from Food and Beverages
125

   128 What Happened to All the Nutrients?
   130 How Do Genetically Modified Foods Cause a Toxic Colon?

133 *How Do Pesticides in Food Cause a Toxic Colon?*
137 *How Do Meat and Dairy Cause a Toxic Colon?*
146 *How Does Soy Cause a Toxic Colon?*
148 *How Does White Flour Cause a Toxic Colon?*
150 *How Does Table Salt Cause a Toxic Colon?*
152 *How Does Monosodium Glutamate Cause a Toxic Colon?*
155 *Cooking Food the Wrong Way!*
159 *Eliminating Intestinal Toxins from Beverages*
161 *How Does Refined Sugar Cause a Toxic Colon?*
165 *Colon Toxins from Artificial Sweeteners*
169 *How Does Caffeine Affect My Colon?*
172 *How Does Alcohol Cause Colon Toxins?*

CHAPTER 8
How to Reduce Intestinal Toxins from Air and Water
179

181 *How Can Air Cause A Toxic Colon?*
183 *How Do Chemical Toxins Present an Indoor Air Hazard?*
187 *Toxins from Biological Contaminants in the Air*
195 *Are You Suffering From Sick Building Syndrome?*
198 *How To Eliminate Intestinal Toxins from Water*
210 *Does a Solution Exist?*

CHAPTER 9
How to Reduce Intestinal Toxins from Drugs and Stress
215

218 *Aren't Prescription Drugs Supposed to Fix What's Wrong with You?*
219 *Can Antibiotics Damage My Colon?*
220 *Are Vaccinations Bad for the Colon?*
224 *How Does Stress Affect My Colon?*

CHAPTER 10
How to Reduce Intestinal Toxins from Heavy Metals & Radiation
235

237 *Intestinal Toxins from Mercury*
240 *Intestinal Toxins from Aluminum*
242 *Intestinal Toxins from Lead*

- 244 Intestinal Toxins from Cadmium
- 245 How Can I Protect Myself from Toxic Heavy Metals?
- 247 Eliminating Intestinal Toxins from Radiation
- 255 Toxic Effects of Geopathic Stress
- 256 How Do I Protect Myself from Radiation?

CHAPTER 11
How to Reduce Intestinal Toxins from Parasites
263

- 264 Intestinal Parasites
- 271 Parasitic Worms That Can Invade the Colon
- 278 How Does Candida Affect My Colon?
- 279 What Bacteria and Viruses are Toxic to My Colon?
- 284 How Do I Avoid These Harmful Organisms?

CHAPTER 12
Liver and Gallbladder Cleansing, Parasite Cleansing, and Heavy Metal Cleansing
289

- 290 Dr. Group's 4-Step Body Cleanse
- 291 Dr. Group's Liver/Gallbladder Cleanse
- 299 Dr. Group's Harmful Organism Cleanse
- 303 Dr. Group's Heavy Metal Cleanse
- 313 Dr. Group's Closing Statements

RESOURCES
317

APPENDIX
365

- 365 Appendix A–Health Questionnaire
- 381 Appendix B–Illustrations

BIBLIOGRAPHY
387

Acknowledgements

I WANT TO THANK YOU FIRST AND FOREMOST AND I DEDICATE THIS BOOK TO YOU!!

If it were not for you this book probably would not have been written, my inspiration and years of knowledge comes from knowing I am helping people everyday. You! are my inspiration and motivation and you are my mentor. So thank you.

There are too many people in my life who have supported me, believed in me, gave me hope, and shared with me information that has literally changed my life. This list would be extremely long and I am limited for space so thanks to everyone who continues to be a part of my life. I really appreciate you believing in me and supporting me over the years. You all know who you are. Thank You, Thank You, Thank You!!!

A special Thanks to my Immediate Family:
My Mom and Dad in the heavens above, my lovely wife Dr. Daniela Group, my newborn organic son Edward IV, Dr. Thetis Group, Dr. Joan Roberts, Dr. Jon Group and Family, Majka (Volim te puno), Tea and Jon Pollock and my favorite nephew Luka. I love you and thank you for all of your support!

Last but Not Least:
The Global Healing Center Family of Employees: Thank you for your commitment to excellence, all of your ideas and effort day in and day out. For helping people everyday recapture their health. For believing and supporting my ideas and vision and making this company successful in making the world a healthier place to live!

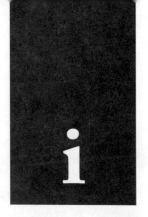

INTRODUCTION

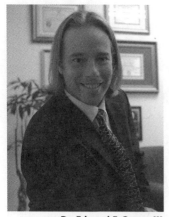

Dr. Edward F. Group III,
DC, ND, DACBN

Over the years, I've gathered a wealth of alternative healing knowledge from both my clinical practice and extensive research on preventing and eliminating disease. I wrote this book to share that information with everyone. Let's face it—the current healthcare systems are not working and the incidence of disease is climbing at an alarming rate. I also want to expose to you the hidden truths behind the medical industry, such as how modern medicine treats just the symptoms of disease and not the root causes.

The great and dark secret of the medical industry is that it's designed to keep you from becoming well. Think about it—how can they stay in business making billions of dollars each year if they actually cured diseases and ended health-related suffering? They know as well as I do—all disease begins by the accumulation of toxins in the body and living in a toxic environment. Every harmful toxin you absorb into your body gets there either through skin contact, air, or by ingesting it directly. I estimate over 90% of all the toxins you take in enter through the intestinal lining! This means disease starts in the digestive tract and *health begins* in the digestive tract.

I feel it's my purpose in life to teach you how critical it is to detoxify your body on the inside as well as the outside. Regardless of what the medical industry tries to teach you through misinformation and misdirection, your body already possesses the God given powers it needs to cure any ailment and disease; but you must learn how to activate your self-healing mechanism. Internal purification is the first, crucial step towards achieving maximum health and vitality. By cleansing your body on a regular basis and eliminating as many toxins as possible from your environment, your body can begin to heal itself, prevent disease, and become stronger and more resilient than you ever dreamed possible!

We've all been taught to take some kind of drug or undergo surgery to fix what ails us. It's just not true! Everyone can take control of their own health once they know how. I truly desire to help society achieve a healthy environment with healthy people enjoying their lives, and I know this is possible by following the secrets I reveal to you in this book.

I am so passionate about what I do because I know cleansing works 100% of the time! I have personally witnessed people eliminating practically every disease from their bodies and regaining superior health after thoroughly cleansing internally and also detoxifying the environments in which they live. I have discovered the ultimate form of happiness by sharing this information and striving to make a real difference in the world. I constantly dream of changing the quality of life for all of us by revealing this valuable information.

The purpose of this book is to give you the tools you need to make it happen—to live a long, healthy, and happy life. I firmly believe—the real definition of a doctor should be one who teaches, not one who prescribes. This is my gift to each and every one of you!

Enjoy,
Dr. Edward Group III, DC, ND, DACBN

PART 1
HOW DISEASE STARTS AND HEALTH BEGINS IN THE COLON

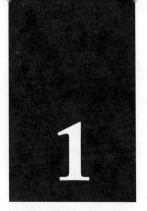

CHAPTER ONE

THE SECRET TO HEALTH

Do you really want to know the single biggest reason why billions of people are suffering from poor health? The answer is right before your eyes!

I am really excited to share with you my conclusions from many years of research. I recently revealed one of the most overlooked and suppressed health secrets in the world (at the *Ninth International Conference on Science and Consciousness* in Santa Fe, New Mexico) at a gathering of international scientists and natural healthcare practitioners as well as medical doctors.

Tragically, this information has been withheld from the general public and has not been included as a part of standard medical training. After years of research, I have finally pieced everything together and I am confident this information is the key to preventing disease and healing the body naturally.

How do I know the answer for reducing and preventing disease?

I have focused on internal body cleansing with my patients my entire career, and I have witnessed the prevention or outright elimination of practically every disease. We always look to science for answers when the explanation is usually quite simple and staring us in the face.

I am excited about sharing this ground-breaking information with you because I know you truly want to maximize your health and help your friends and family regain their wellbeing and prevent disease. I have committed my life to helping as many people as I can and I hope you will do the same. The time has come to get this information out to the public.

This information is for YOU! Though you may have been taught to believe otherwise, you CAN begin taking responsibility for your own health today.

SO WHAT IS THIS SECRET TO HEALTH?

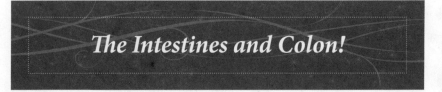

The Intestines and Colon!

Did you know most disease-causing toxins enter the body through the intestines?

The intestines are the first point of attack for virtually all disease-causing agents. These toxins make their way into the bloodstream, subsequently causing blood toxemia or congestive toxicosis, overworking the liver,

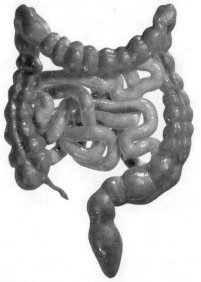

Fig. I: Healthy Colon

and then infiltrating every type of tissue. This process is the origin of the "dis-ease" mechanism. A small amount of toxins enter through the skin and lungs via direct contact and respiration respectively.

Parasites, toxins from food, toxins from water, toxins from heavy metals, toxins from milk, soft drinks, coffee, alcohol, drugs, and everything else you ingest enter the body through the intestinal lining.

The intestinal lining is exposed to millions of toxins every day!

Even toxins from the air you breathe pass through the intestines. These toxins become caught in the mucous linings of the mouth or nasal passages and then drain into the stomach, eventually making their way into the intestines.

Toxic intestines are simply not able to function properly because they are inhibited by layers of accumulated, impacted waste material. This creates a narrowed passageway leading to constipation and other bowel problems. Constipation, as you know, makes having regular bowel movements difficult and leads to further impaction. If toxins are not eliminated from the intestines on a regular basis, they leach back into the bloodstream through what is called "leaky gut syndrome" where they can ultimately cause disease.

Why Has This Been Kept a "Secret"?

Perhaps "secret" isn't the most accurate word. Plain "lack of knowledge" might be a better choice. Ask any doctor to explain the role of the intestines and how they function in the body and I guarantee they will not be able to give you a definitive answer. Why is this? The answer is simple ...

Doctors Are Not Being Taught to <u>Prevent</u> Disease!

If preventative measures and cleansing were taught in medical schools, many diseases we take for granted would simply cease to exist. The pharmaceutical industry, government-funded medical research, and virtual armies of around-the-clock medical staff would be unnecessary if people discovered all they had to do to achieve optimal health was just keep their intestines, liver, body, and living environment clean. What we're really talking about is the loss of hundreds of billions of dollars in annual healthcare revenue![1]

Medical Science Can Explain the Function of Every Organ In the Body Except . . . the Appendix?

Sound strange? Well, why do you think so many people have their appendix removed? Doctors still don't know what the appendix is, much less what it does. Standard treatment methods as taught in medical schools dictate removing the appendix whenever it becomes inflamed. Why? The medical industry realizes a simple truth—without your appendix, you are destined for illness so doctors can prescribe you more drugs, perform more unnecessary surgeries, or (even worse) treat you with deadly radiation as a "cure" that's definitely worse than the disease.

So why is the appendix so important anyway? Here's my theory: The appendix is located at the juncture of the small and large intestines and acts as a body regulator and communicator. The appendix monitors internal pH, the toxic load present, and the opening and closing of the ileocecal valve, plus it sends messages to the immune system regarding activity in the bowel.

The appendix is made up of lymphoid tissue (immune cells) and it regulates lymphatic, exocrine, endocrine, and neuromuscular functions. The appendix basically acts as a microcomputer relay station for the body. You might be wondering—why would the body's regulatory computer be located in the colon of all places? My answer is—why wouldn't it be? The intestinal tract is the first place everything enters our bodies! **It has been estimated more than 200,000 appendices are removed in the United States each year![2]**

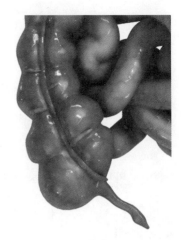

Fig. II: Appendix

All too often, the digestive system and the colon in particular have the status of being "second-class organs" because we're embarrassed about their function—eliminating waste. Consider for a moment just how important these components are in the grand scheme of biology—the intestines are the first exposure point and thus the first line of defense against environmental toxins to which we expose ourselves daily.

Imagine what would happen if you never cleaned your house, never took out the garbage, never vacuumed your car, or never took a shower. What would happen to your body (or your social life for that matter) after 10 years of wallowing in filth? Your body would likely be repellent and disgusting beyond belief.

Guess what? If you ignore your colon for ten years (or twenty or thirty), the same pollution and damage can happen on the inside of your body! I have spent years tracing the root causes of disease. Although everyone talks about toxic overload, no one is focusing on the real problem—where that overload takes place.

What Happens When You Have a Toxic Intestine, Colon, or Liver?

I mention the liver at this point because, after years of toxic buildup, the liver takes quite a beating and must be cleansed regularly just like your skin, house, or car. However, the intestinal tract is the first line of defense in the body. If toxins never infiltrate into the bloodstream from the intestines in the first place, the liver can function in its normal capacity.

When I had my natural health practice, I took on the hardest cancer and degenerative disease cases I could find because I loved the challenge. Patients would sometimes ask me during the initial consultation, "What are you going to do for me that all the other doctors couldn't do?"

I said to them, "Let me ask you a question . . . what did all the other doctors do to cleanse or detoxify your body before giving you bottles of prescription medications (or bags of supplements)?" Practically every one of them would respond with confusion, "Cleanse? What is that?" Well, I didn't just tell them ...

I Showed My Patients the Positive Effect Cleansing Could Have on Their Health!

These men and women were amazed–after a few months of cleansing, half their symptoms were already gone . . . and we hadn't even started addressing their condition yet! These results were just from the cleansing regimens I advised! I then explained to them I don't actually "heal" anyone. True healing takes place from within. It's your responsibility to heal yourself.

As a Doctor, It is My Responsibility and Moral Obligation to Teach You <u>How</u> to Heal Yourself!

Now, I tell people to start with the 6-Day Oxygen Colon Cleanse followed by three consecutive Liver/Gallbladder Cleanses, plus the Harmful Organism Cleanse and Heavy Metal Cleanse. I phase in their unique supplement regimen only after the first colon and liver cleanses are complete. After the initial cleansing of these organs, their bodies are ready to begin the natural healing process.

People may have a shopping list of symptoms, but doctors are not finding and certainly not treating the root causes of disease! Most symptoms will disappear after a successful program of internal cleansing.

You can give people the finest quality, wildcrafted, super-organic health supplements in the world until you are blue in the face, but you are still not addressing the core of their problem. Toxic overload results from a lack of internal cleansing!

What people do not realize is they need to cleanse their intestines on a regular basis as part of an ongoing health routine. *It is generally accepted that bowel movement frequency can range from 3 per day to 3 per week, but some people have just 2 per week or fewer.* Can you imagine the fermentation, putrefaction, rancidity, and sheer amount of toxins leaking into the bloodstream from a polluted colon that produces only two bowel movements a week?

A healthy person should have three to four bowel movements daily. Don't think so? This principle can be demonstrated by the animal kingdom. For every meal consumed, birds, fish, insects, and mammals have corresponding bowel movements.

Even the Earth cleanses itself regularly with rain, snow melt-off, wind, volcanic eruptions, lightning etc. Human beings should be no different. We should be having three to four normal bowel movements daily and cleansing regularly.

A healthy bowel transit time should be 12 to 18 hours. The average transit time in Western countries is at least twice that—38 hours or more![3]

It absolutely amazes me that we supposedly have the best medical researchers in the world and no one has made the connection between bowel transit time and the incidence of disease and digestive health in particular! "An assessment of colonic transit time enables the healthcare provider to better understand the rate of stool movement through the colon …" since, obviously, disease or impairment within the digestive system can lead to reduced efficiency.[4] In other words, the slowing down of transit time can indicate the onset of constipation or further bowel disease.

Constipation and Other Digestive Disorders Affect 1 out of 5 People in America![5]

Most doctors respond to constipation by recommending a laxative, which is essentially a drug. Laxative sales in the last four years alone exceeded $2.7 billion.[6] One can easily conclude constipation (ironically, often drug-induced) is a very serious health concern in the United States. As westernized society continues to spread, digestive disorders are becoming prevalent in many other countries as well.

So what is the response to digestive disease by the pharmaceutical companies? These companies depend on product longevity so they develop and patent laxatives which cause even further bowel damage so they can keep selling you their "treatment." If they actually cured anything, these companies would go out of business because they wouldn't be needed anymore.

This obvious conflict between eliminating disease and continued profit makes me wonder if that's the reason why most pharmaceutical drugs list "constipation" as a major side effect. You take something to treat your pain, high blood pressure, or arthritis and you end up needing laxatives to treat the accompanying constipation. We have "lemon" laws to protect consumers from deceptive auto salesmen but it's apparently an accepted practice for drug manufacturers to grow rich from your misery. These companies sell you even more drugs instead of fixing what's wrong by addressing the root cause of your problem.

The key to renewed health is obviously to eliminate as many toxins as you can from your environment on a daily basis (see Part II—*How to Live in a Green, Toxin Free Environment*) before they even reach your intestines. Let's face one of the main problems though—addiction!

How Many People Do You Know Who Would Be Willing to Give Up Their:

- Choice cuts of meat (steak, veal, brisket, pork)
- Convenient fast foods (pizza, burgers, tacos, fried chicken)
- Morning-motivating coffee (lattés, cappuccino, espresso)
- Delicious dairy (milk, butter, cheese, ice-cream)
- "Social lubricant" alcohol (beer, wine, mixed drinks)
- Soft drinks, energy drinks, diet drinks, and fruit flavored drinks
- Smile-giving sugar (chocolate, cake, pie, candy-bars)
- White flour (tortillas, "enriched" wheat and white bread, doughnuts)
- And everything else that tastes good but is really bad for us

And what about all of the depression, anxiety, fear, negative belief patterns, and learned behaviors that cause disease? From where do you think these negative emotions originate?

Toxins leaking into our bodies from the intestines! These chemicals disrupt sensitive biochemical and hormonal balances by altering the electrical signals in the water within blood and our living cells.

This disruption in the brain can cause depression, mood disorders, and other emotional disturbances. Once people start cleansing internally, emotional disorders often go away. Do you ever go about your day feeling like you're in a fog, like everything is slightly out of focus or you can't concentrate like you used to? This perpetual haze isn't caused by just the natural aging process. Your mental clarity can be affected by the toxic substances you consume.

> **TO RAISE THE CONSCIOUSNESS OF THE PLANET AND TO ACHIEVE TRUE SPIRITUALITY, OUR BODIES NEED TO BE PURE!**

Think about the last time you felt really healthy. Take a moment to remember how your mind and body and spirit felt. You probably were self-confident and eager to face the day because you looked and felt *great*. You actually loved yourself and desired to experience life in its rich variety. You enjoyed your connections with other people in your life, your community, and the larger world. Well, I assure you that if you take to heart and practice the methods that I detail in this book, you can feel that way again. When you cleanse your body regularly, and deal with bad health habits generally, you can regain your self-confidence and sense of self and renewed hope for the future. You can believe again that you are capable of achieving anything you put your mind to. This encourages success in anything you manifest through your thoughts and actions. No more secrets. To be happy and healthy, you must be clean inside and out! So let's move on to Chapter 2 and start learning about the intestinal tract.

2

CHAPTER TWO

WHAT IS A TOXIC COLON?

Let's pretend that your body is a car. Every 3,000 miles or so you need to have your oil and filters changed because they've become caked with sticky black grunge from your engine. This buildup of sludge forces your engine to work harder to keep the car moving. All this extra work increases the wear and tear on your engine, and if something isn't done about it, eventually your engine will break down.

Most of us drive our cars for only a few hours each day, so we need to have the oil changed just once every two to three months. Your body, on the other hand, is working 24 hours a day and most of us go years without cleansing the insides of our bodies.

In many ways, your colon is like the exhaust pipe of a car. The gas in the fuel tank is sucked into the engine where it's mixed with air and fire to combust. This controlled explosion moves the pistons that create the energy to make the tires turn. This is a complicated process requiring a near perfect balance of various mechanical, electrical, and chemical reactions. These processes create certain byproducts or toxic residue. In the case of your car, those toxins are exhaust emissions.

Your body works in much the same way. The foods you eat are pumped from your stomach into your intestines where they are broken down to create the energy that keeps you moving. The foods we fuel our bodies with also create byproducts. If the intestines are functioning properly, these byproducts are expelled two to four times a day through regular bowel movements.

When your car's engine isn't running smoothly and its exhaust pipe becomes congested with polluted gunk, it backfires. So what do you think happens to your body when your colon becomes congested with its own kind of gunk?

Have you ever seen a rusted-out exhaust pipe with holes in it? Besides making it difficult to pass an emissions test, these holes can allow toxic exhaust fumes to leak into the passenger area of your car. With time, your colon can also develop holes. These holes allow toxins to leak into your bloodstream. Eventually, these toxins creep into other organs and bodily tissues where they fester and cause disease.

Over the last 100 years, mankind has polluted the air, the food, the water, and practically everything else we've been able to get our hands on. We watch all of these things occurring and still seem to think, "It doesn't concern me."

Well, think again. Our bodies are absorbing this toxic pollution, and the harsh reality is—approximately one out of every thirty people in the United States is developing some form of cancer during their lifetime (based on 2004 updated data).[7] Today we are faced with more disease than ever before and it keeps getting worse.

It may seem hard to believe, but all of the toxins discussed in this book enter the body through the mouth, nose, or skin, and they are absorbed directly through the intestines. Most people think the toxins they consume affect only their liver or kidneys, but that isn't the whole truth. Even though these organs process or filter as many toxins as they can, they eventually become overworked and overwhelmed.

Normally, the liver tries to convert substances it receives from the digestive system into nutrients we can use. The problem is—both the liver and intestines are faced with more toxins now than they can possibly handle. These organs quickly become caught in a vicious cycle of passing toxins back and forth. All of our organs are dangerously overworked, but moreso the intestines.

Before going any further, I'd like to make something clear—for ease of reading, I will often be referring to the "colon" and "intestines" as one entity. *Health Begins in the Colon* certainly describes colon cleansing, but just focusing on the colon without concentrating on the full intestinal tract would be addressing only half the problem. The small intestine and the colon (large intestine) must be cleansed regularly for you to achieve better health.

Another word you're going to see used frequently is "toxin". By strict definition, a toxin is any substance of organic origin that is damaging to living tissue. For the sake of simplicity, we'll be using "toxin" generically to mean any foreign substance wreaking havoc on your health once it's inside your body. In the end, whether we're talking about airborne pollutants from a refinery or yeast overgrowth in your intestines, the results are the same—a toxic colon and body.

A general understanding of the inner workings of the colon and its processes is necessary for you to learn how to improve your intestinal health. Now, let's begin a brief overview of the anatomy and physiology of the colon.

What Exactly Does the Colon Do?

The colon, or large intestine, is one of the primary components of your digestive system. It's made up of basically the same types of tissue found in your throat, stomach, and small intestines, but the colon has a few unique characteristics that set it apart from the rest of the digestive tract. For one thing, no part of the large intestine produces digestive enzymes. That task is left entirely to the small intestine.

The colon is divided into four parts—the Ascending colon, the Transverse colon, the Descending colon, and the Sigmoid colon. Please refer to the image below.

After leaving the small intestines, waste enters the ascending colon on the right side of the abdomen. The ascending colon moves waste upwards to the transverse colon (spanning the gap to the descending

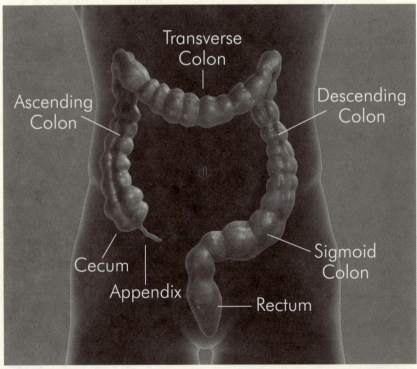

Fig. III: Anatomy of the Colon

colon) which in turn carries waste down through the sigmoid colon and out through the rectum.

Most of the vitamins and nutrients our bodies receive from the foods we eat have already been absorbed by the small intestines before reaching the colon. The colon's primary job is absorbing the left over water to condense soft byproducts into solid waste. The colon also takes in select water-tied nutrients such as electrolytes. The colon and small intestine can also absorb dangerous toxins and, unfortunately, these toxins are the root cause of most degenerative disease.

A healthy colon is essential for your overall wellbeing. The colon is more than just a tube for the food you eat to pass through on its way out; it's a key part of the digestive process. When the colon stops functioning properly, digestion becomes disrupted and the essential vitamins, minerals, and other nutrients your body depends on to grow and thrive are no longer absorbed. An unhealthy colon is also less able to expel toxins.

What Causes the Colon to Malfunction in the First Place?

The foods we eat obviously have a lot to do with keeping our colons healthy, but if maintaining our colons is as easy as making a few small changes to our dietary habits, why does the incidence of disease continue to skyrocket even among people with otherwise healthy diets? Well, the real problem is our constant exposure to everyday toxins.

Day-in and day-out, we're drowning in a sea of toxic substances our bodies aren't designed to handle. We eat chemically tainted food and drink contaminated water and beverages. We breathe polluted smog instead of oxygen-rich air. When we finally notice our bodies beginning to break down, most people go to a medical doctor for help.

These doctors prescribe synthetic drugs that add to the problem. Drugs may help alleviate the symptoms, but they do nothing to treat the root cause of the disease.

> **DEFINITION**
>
> **Leaky Gut Syndrome:** The formation of microscopic holes in the intestinal lining (caused by prescription drugs, poor diet, toxic materials, etc.) leading to increased permeability allowing food particles, toxins, parasites, and heavy metals to enter the bloodstream.
>
> **Degenerative Disease:** A state of disease in which the affected tissue progressively deteriorates over time.

Unbelievably, nearly every disease known to humanity is caused, triggered, or amplified by a toxic colon. As I explained in Chapter 1, nearly every toxin entering the body passes through the intestinal tract. Toxins are not always expelled in a timely manner either. These toxins become trapped in intestinal mucous tissues, thus crippling the entire digestive system. Next, these toxins leak their way back into the body, weakening it and further slowing down intestinal processing.

Unfortunately, the vast majority of the medical establishment still fails to accept the importance of maintaining a clean colon for personal health. Are you beginning to see a pattern emerge? If toxins are not eliminated from the colon on a regular basis, they leak into the bloodstream through what is termed "**leaky gut syndrome**,"[8] and cause **degenerative diseases** throughout the body.

Okay, so where exactly do all of these toxins originate? More importantly, what can we do to prevent toxicity and maintain our precious health? You already know our environment is in pretty bad shape, but do you know why toxins are hurting us or how they're doing it?

An unhealthy living environment leads to disease! Very few of us take proactive steps to shield our bodies from toxins, much less fight against the industries responsible for creating them in the first place. To fully grasp the effects of toxins in your body, you must first understand the unique factors of your body. How healthy are the foods you eat? Do you exercise each day? How high is your personal toxin threshold?

How Clogged Are Our Colons?

More than sixty million people in the United States are overweight to some degree.[9] I'd say that's pretty clogged. According to the Centers for Disease Control and Prevention, "Results from the 2003-2004 Na-

Leaky Gut Syndrome

ANATOMICAL OVERVIEW:

Sectional view of the colon displaying shape and texture of villi densely lining the interior surface.

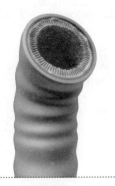

MAGNIFIED VIEW:

A single villus from the colon wall contains a complex network of capillaries for distributing nutrients into the bloodstream.

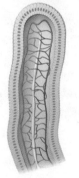

MICROSCOPIC VIEW:

The outer sheath of a villus is in turn lined with tiny epithelial cells through which toxins may enter the bloodstream and cause disease.

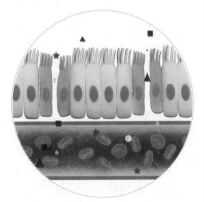

▲ = Nutrients
★ = Heavy Metals/Toxic Chemicals
● = Undigested Food Particles
■ = Parasites

Fig. IV

> **DEFINITION**
>
> ***Impacted waste:***
> The accumulation of hard compacted fecal matter from years of poor dietary habits and toxic buildup. This waste matter adheres to the walls of the intestines and is not eliminated during regular bowel movements.

tional Health and Nutrition Examination Survey (NHANES) … indicate that an estimated 66 percent of U.S. adults are either overweight or obese."[10] Poor adult health can often be traced to unhealthful habits developed during childhood.

What do these findings tell us? Obviously, we are raising obese children that become obese adults; but if we read between the lines, they also tell us generations of Americans are spending their entire lives facing constipation. Without intervention, obesity can become a lifelong problem. We can put an end to this crisis and prevent children from becoming obese by teaching them about proper diet and exercise.

What does any of that have to do with a toxic colon? This trend towards increased body fat might not seem closely related to colon toxicity, but it helps illustrate the common causes of colon toxicity—poor diet, lack of exercise, and a toxic living environment.

A well-balanced diet is essential to staying lean, healthy, and toxin-free, but a sudden spike on the bathroom scale may have less to do with what goes into your body than with what comes out of it (or in this case, what doesn't). Often, it's the same fatty foods that are synonymous with an increase in weight that lead to clogged colons.

Hardened waste that obstructs bowel activity can also contribute to obesity. Perhaps you've heard the myth that John Wayne had over 40 pounds of **impacted waste** in his colon at the time of his death. In truth, the average American probably has several pounds of hard, compacted fecal matter caked along the sides of their bowels by the time they're 30 years old.

That's years worth of toxins festering away inside the body. If healthy, consistent bowel movements and regular colon cleansing had eliminated the bulk of these toxins, this situation could have been prevented. Toxic residue accumulates over time and can lead to swelling in the walls of the large intestine. This is just one of the more obvious symptoms of "bowel toxemia" or a **toxic colon**.

It's easy to see the differences between the two pictures below. The colon on the left is obviously healthy and full of life. Unfortunately, the average colon looks a lot more like the disease-ridden image on the right.

> **DEFINITION**
>
> *Toxic Colon:*
> A colon that has been damaged by toxic substances causing injury or illness.

Going to the bathroom when you need to is one of the most important things you can do to help maintain your health. Many people are so busy they simply won't take the time to have a bowel movement when the urge strikes. Some people prefer to have bowel movements only at home and will go to great lengths to avoid using a public restroom. If the delay is too long or too frequent, ignoring the urge to "go" can lead to constipation and fecal compaction, both of which contribute to toxic buildup in the colon.

Constipation and fecal impaction can cause stool transit time to slow down. "Transit time" is basically the time it takes our bodies to process and pass waste. If undigested food remains in the body too long, proteins putrefy, carbohydrates ferment, and fats turn rancid. This changes the compounds in the food so they become harmful instead of beneficial.

Normal Healthy Colon   **Unhealthy Toxic Colon**

Fig. V: Comparison of Healthy and Unhealthy Colons

This rotten food collects inside the colon, making regular bowel movements increasingly difficult.

Have you ever noticed that some people who smoke, drink, and never exercise still live long, disease-free lives while others who make healthy choices and practice balanced, vegetarian diets develop illnesses? It doesn't make sense, does it?

Everyone has their own tolerances for chemicals and other substances entering the body that are dependent on lifestyle, environmental exposure, stress levels, and even genetics. This is known as the body's "toxic threshold" or the amount of toxic abuse the body can handle on a daily basis before it starts to break down.

To provide you an example of how many factors discussed in this book contribute to a toxic colon and the importance of regular intestinal cleansing, I've created a list of daily toxin-exposure examples. There's no way to know exactly how many toxins from each category you're taking in each day, but this gives you an idea of the risk factors and toxins from each category.

Depending on your everyday environmental and personal health choices, these numbers could be greater or less than the examples provided.

Examples of Potential Daily Toxin Intake

Let's assume your body can handle only 1 million toxins every 24 hours before it's overloaded.

Every 24 hours, you may consume the following amounts of toxins in an average lifestyle:

Toxins from Food: 325,000
White flour, sugar in desserts, hormones and antibiotics, soy, pesticides, genetically modified foods, MSG, hydrogenated oils, fast foods and cooked, boxed, canned, processed foods, etc.

Toxins from Beverages: 160,000
Pasteurized milk, soft drinks, diet colas, "energy" (highly caffeinated)

drinks, sports drinks, juice concentrates, coffee, alcohol, refined sugars, artificial sweeteners, artificial coloring, etc.

Toxins from Air: 200,000
Fossil fuels, benzene, smoke, chemtrail residue, paint fumes, carpet outgassing, pet dander, mold and mildew, dust mites, air fresheners, cleaning supplies, etc.

Toxins from Water: 150,000
Arsenic, fluoride, chlorine, prescription drug residue, pesticides, rocket fuel (perchlorate), Bisphenol-A (toxin used in making plastic water bottles), C_8 (the chemical used to make Teflon®[11]), bacteria, parasites, etc.

Toxins from Prescription Drugs: 180,000
Aluminum, mercury, chemotherapy, left-over animal parts from meat processing plants, synthetic chemicals, liver toxic glues, fillers, binders, artificial colorings, spermicides, synthetic hormones, vaccines, etc.

Toxins from Microbes (Parasites): 525,000
Bacteria, yeast, fungus, worms, amoebas, and viruses all feed off a host organism (you in this case). These organisms consume your vital nutrients and then deposit waste matter (massive amounts of harmful acids and toxins) in your system.

Toxins from Physical / Emotional Stress: 200,000
Depression, anxiety, fear, and other negative emotions cause the body to over-produce stress hormones and other compounds to fight these conditions. This is dangerous because the body damages itself in the process.

Toxins from Heavy Metals: 130,000
Cookware, deodorant, chemically poisoned fish, mercury dental fillings, cosmetics, aluminum cans, food, water, light bulbs, many herbal supplements, toothpaste, vaccines, household and automobile paints, etc.

Toxins from Radiation: (Causes Cell Damage and Death): 230,000
Microwave cooking, X-rays, fault lines (geopathic stress), power lines, cellphones, computers, household appliances, fluorescent lighting, hair dryers, irradiated foods, etc.

Total: 2,100,000 toxins every 24 hours—more than twice what I've proposed as a maximum tolerance!

This may seem like an enormous number of toxins, but a single bag of a synthetic sugar substitute can contain over ten thousand toxic molecules in the form of artificial ingredients! Don't worry, I will describe each type of toxin in greater detail in Chapters 7 through 11, and I'll tell you exactly how to either replace or eliminate these toxic substances from your diet and environment.

If your body can handle only 1 million toxins, but you are exposed to over 2.1 million toxins each day, your body has to work extra hard, expend valuable energy, and process or store these compounds to get them out of the way. Your body is losing vital energy all the time from trying to detoxify and flush out these substances!

Now can you see what's happening inside your body every day?

I like to give the example of one million but this is actually a very low estimate. Your intestinal lining is directly exposed to these toxins every day and, if these toxins are not eliminated, they can leak into the bloodstream initiating the disease process.

In *Part II—How to Live in a Green, Toxin Free Environment*, I'm going to explain to you how disease originates from a toxic colon and I'm going to go over some shocking statistics, but my job is to teach you how to prevent disease, how to clean the intestines and body properly, and how to activate your body's self-healing mechanism. I believe people need to know how to address and eliminate the root cause of their health problems as well as addressing any current symptoms they may have.

We have other options available to us besides total reliance on the medical system. We do not need a prescription drug or surgery to fix everything. Drugs and surgeries do not address the root cause of the condition. That's why I wrote this book, so you can understand why we're dealing with so many degenerative diseases and toxic colons today. It's a combination of factors directly related to the environment to which you expose yourself. It's not just one particular toxin (such as cigarette smoke, alcohol, or fried foods) that causes disease. It's a combination of many different factors caused by too many toxins coming in and not enough going out!

As I have stated before, the colon is the most neglected organ in the body, perhaps due to embarrassment or lack of knowledge regarding its importance in the health hierarchy. Nevertheless, the colon usually does not receive as much attention as other organs in the body. The colon is just as vital to life as the other organs and, in fact, it can be the determining factor between feeling great or living a life filled with illness and fatigue.

If everyone knew that regaining their health was as easy as cleaning their bodies regularly and slowly changing the environments in which they live and work, as a society, we wouldn't need or be dependent upon prescription drugs. This concept probably doesn't sit well with the pharmaceutical industry's moneymaking scheme of addressing only symptoms instead of the root cause of disease!

CHAPTER THREE

CONDITIONS OF A TOXIC COLON

This chapter briefly explains some of the more common conditions caused by the accumulation of toxins in the colon. We've touched on some of these toxins briefly and how they cause disease, but you might be thinking at this point, "There's nothing wrong with my bowel." Most people believe this, but please read on as you may be in for a surprise.

Now you're going to learn exactly what can happen when you don't cleanse your intestines and colon on a regular basis.

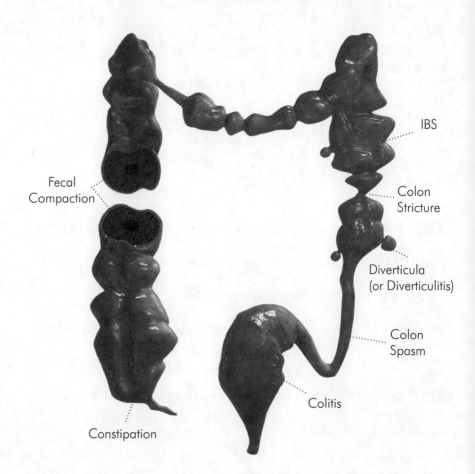

COMMON BOWEL CONDITIONS CAUSED BY EVERYDAY TOXIN EXPOSURE

Constipation: What is it?

Millions of Americans exhibit constipation symptoms ranging from slower than normal transit time to full, chronic constipation on a frequent basis. Personally, I feel the majority of people have clogged colons to some degree. Constipation is so prevalent and widespread it should be listed as an epidemic. Whether you think so or not, you are probably constipated according to the true meaning of the word. The shocking truth is—the medical definition of constipation is just plain wrong!

The Medical Definition of Constipation: The passage of small amounts of hard, dry bowel movements, usually fewer than three times per week.

Like I said in Chapter 1, birds, horses, cows, rabbits, ducks, and anything that lives and eats from the Earth produces multiple bowel movements daily, sometimes more than 10 per day. When is the last time you saw a cow straining in the field or a bird constipated (instead of "decorating" every statue in sight)? Your bowel habits should be no different. We should be having multiple bowel movements daily!

The Real Definition of Constipation: If you are not having a minimum of 2 soft, easy to pass bowel movements daily then you are constipated because waste is accumulating in your system. If your stools are soft, do not have a foul odor, and they are passed easily and frequently (at least 2 times a day), I would say you are not constipated.

Even if you're going pretty regularly, you can still have pounds of hard compacted fecal matter in your intestinal tract. Many people suffering from constipation feel like they have incomplete bowel evacuations and this causes them to strain even more. Straining can lead to anal fissures or hemorrhoids over time. Other symptoms of constipation can include increased bowel sounds, fatigue (from the toxins), bad breath, and skin blemishes.

You might be surprised to learn bad breath is a commonly overlooked symptom of constipation, but it makes perfect sense when you think about it. After all, the mouth and stomach are connected. A digestive tract that's sluggish due to constipation can cause the mouth to have a putrid odor because of gasses rising up from the stomach and lingering in the mouth. Plus, bad breath means your body is trying to tell you something. If you smell this odor, you need to address the root cause by cleansing your system and eliminating toxins from your environment. Your body will always give you signs when something is wrong. You just need to learn how to listen to them.

Skin eruptions or blemishes can also be signs of a colon trying to eliminate toxins. It's true—constipation can cause acne or worsen existing skin problems. Many people fail to understand the skin is a major organ that aids in eliminating waste. If the liver and kidneys become overwhelmed by toxic substances that need to be evacuated from the body, the skin does its very best to help in this effort through sweating.

Individuals who are constipated are typically backed up inside with fecal matter. While it's impossible for the skin to remove fecal matter, the epidermis (the outer layer of the skin) can show symptoms of attempting to rid the body of toxins by breaking out.

Many people ignore their constipation because they have lived with it for so long. These individuals have forgotten what it feels like to be healthy and to have normal bowel movements. Ignoring constipation is not a good idea and doing so can put your health in danger. Living with constipation should never be "acceptable" to anyone. Constipation is one of many precursors for all bowel disorders and other diseases of the body.

Untreated constipation can lead to very serious problems such as bowel obstruction, which is characterized by a tender stomach and vomiting. Ironically, constipation can also lead to episodes of diarrhea. Many people who experience diarrhea don't realize it could be a symptom of constipation. Paradoxical diarrhea occurs when soft or liquid waste matter passes around the impacted matter lodged in the colon. X-rays performed during these stages of constipation can reveal the location of the impacted fecal matter in the bowel, and surgery is sometimes required in cases of severe constipation.

The good news is—by keeping their intestines and colons cleansed, people do not have to suffer from constipation any longer!

How Does Regular Intestinal Cleansing Eliminate Constipation?

- Cleans the encrusted buildup from the walls of the intestinal lining, thereby increasing the absorption of the vital nutrients your body needs
- Helps promote bowel movements that are more frequent
- Helps promote better consistency and volume of stool
- Makes it easier to pass stools without straining
- Greatly reduces the chances of developing constipation-related diseases
- Reduces the number of toxins absorbed into the blood
- Improves bowel transit time (time from eating to elimination)

IBS: What is Irritable Bowel Syndrome?

Irritable Bowel Syndrome affects about 14% of American adults![12]

DEFINITION
Serotonin: a chemical hormone that carries messages from one part of your body to another. Serotonin helps regulate emotions, body temperature, sexuality, appetite, and bowel function.

Irritable Bowel Syndrome (IBS), also called "spastic colon," is characterized by mild but persistent problems in the gut. IBS symptoms may even pose long-term danger to the colon, and IBS can seriously interfere with the everyday lives of people with the condition. In most cases, the triggers and symptoms of IBS can be managed through a combination of dietary and lifestyle improvements along with consistent colon cleansing.

What are the symptoms of IBS?

Abdominal discomfort and bloating are the most commonly reported complaints, but a number of other symptoms are also regularly documented. Some people are chronically constipated and report straining to have a bowel movement. Some people experience diarrhea, which is on the opposite end of the "bowel movement spectrum," and still other people experience alternating bouts of constipation and diarrhea.

Moreover, people with IBS frequently suffer from depression and anxiety, which can worsen their symptoms. Similarly, the symptoms associated with IBS can cause a person to feel depressed and anxious, so the cycle repeats itself.

Did You Know?
Serotonin *is produced and stored within the cells lining the digestive tract. Current research suggests serotonin plays a key role in the motor-sensory and excretory functions of the digestive tract and that damaged receptor sites may contribute to the onset of IBS. In fact, "Serotonin is… a vital link in the brain-gut axis."*[13] *Imbalanced serotonin levels may therefore lead to increased abdominal discomfort and bowel movement difficulty.*

According to medical science, no specific cause of IBS has been identified, although some theories suggest many people with IBS may be overly sensitive to certain substances that do not bother the typical digestive system. Stress, large meals, gas, medicines, certain foods, coffee, milk, and alcohol are some of the many stimuli that can irritate the colon.

I'll let you in on a little secret—you want to know what really causes IBS? (I'm sure you already know by this point.) It's the accumulation and constant bombardment of toxins within your colon!

Who is at risk for IBS?

Irritable Bowel Syndrome occurs about 30% more often in women than in men[14], and it tends to begin in early adulthood. Genetics may play a role since many people who suffer from IBS have relatives that also have IBS.

It can be quite difficult to diagnose this condition because there are no indications presented during a standard colon examination. Instead, doctors are forced to rely entirely upon the medical history provided by the patient. Not everyone who has IBS seeks treatment due to embarrassment, economic difficulties (no insurance), lack of health education, etc. and this is one of the most often misdiagnosed conditions. "One challenge of population-based IBS studies is ensuring that IBS is accurately diagnosed using specific, validated criteria, rather than the clinical judgement of health care professionals."[15]

How Does Regular Colon Cleansing Help Relieve and Prevent IBS?

- Eliminates built up toxins and rids the intestinal walls of yeast and harmful bacteria (this sets the stage for rebalancing your intestinal flora with beneficial bacteria). People with IBS lack beneficial Probiotic bacteria in their bowels

- Helps relieve stress and anxiety, which contribute to flare-ups of IBS

- Helps calm the irritated and overactive nerves in the intestinal tract thereby reducing inflammation associated with IBS
- Decreases transit time to reduce the constant irritation of the bowel lining
- Helps relieve abdominal cramping, bloating, gas, and pain associated with IBS

Diverticular Disease: What Is It?

As we age, the lining of our intestines becomes thin and loses elasticity. Small pouches of tissue known as diverticula bulge through these weak areas. Diverticula range in diameter from 5 to more than 20 millimeters. Nearly one-third of adult Americans have at least a few of these pouches in their intestines, and some studies estimate as much as sixty percent of the elderly population has them.[16] The condition of having these small pouches is referred to as Diverticulosis.

For the most part, Diverticulosis goes unnoticed. But in about one-fifth of the cases, the pouches become irritated or infected and this is referred to as Diverticulitis. The infected pouches can make a bowel movement very painful, which can lead to chronic constipation and other health complications.

DOCTOR'S NOTE:

In the United States alone, Diverticular disease accounts for over a million physician office and hospital visits each year.[17]

What are the symptoms of Diverticular Disease?

Many people experience no symptoms whatsoever with Diverticulosis, but some have reported mild cramps, constipation, and bloating. Diverticulitis, on the other hand, is characterized by abdominal pain (especially along the left side), cramping, constipation, fever, nausea,

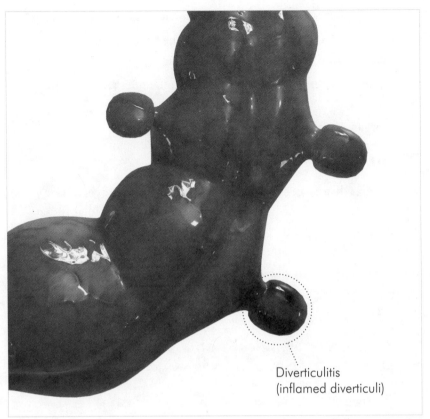

Fig. VI: Diverticula

vomiting, and chills.

Since these symptoms are associated with a number of other intestinal conditions, Diverticular disease can be difficult to diagnose. To make a prognosis, a doctor will first ask a series of questions about the patient's bowel habits, diet, and other risk factors. A digital rectal examination may also be performed. Other methods include X-rays, ultrasound, CT scanning, colonoscopy, and sigmoidoscopy.

Untreated, the disease can also lead to a number of serious complications, most of which arise when a portion of the colon wall becomes torn or perforated. Because of this tearing, toxic waste matter can leak from the intestines into the abdominal cavity and may cause serious health problems including:

- **Abscesses**—Infections in the abdomen that become "walled off"
- **Peritonitis**—A painful infection of the abdominal cavity that is can be life threatening
- **Obstructions**—Physical blockages in the intestines
- **Fistulas**—A connection between two organs or between an organ and the skin

Who is at risk for Diverticular Disease?

Diverticular disease becomes more common as people age. In fact, almost 70 percent of the population will develop Diverticular disease by the age of 85.[18] Again, the constant bombardment of colon toxins (especially from food) contributes to an increased risk for developing this condition.

How Does Regular Colon Cleansing Prevent and Relieve Symptoms of Diverticular Disease?

- Eliminates built up toxins which may be stored in Diverticular pouches
- Rids the intestinal walls of the harmful bacteria and yeast causing Diverticulitis (infection and inflammation)
- Prevents the diverticuli from becoming infected and swollen
- Helps relieve constipation (which contributes to the development of Diverticular Disease)
- Strengthens the intestinal walls to prevent thinning, weakening, and bulging
- Decreases transit time, thereby reducing exposure of the bowel lining to toxic irritants
- Helps restore proper bowel function, which also lowers the chances of developing Diverticulitis
- Encourages growth of beneficial bacteria

Celiac Disease: What Is It?

At least 2 ¼ million people in the U.S. have Celiac disease (CD) and this number continues to rise.[19]

> **DEFINITION**
>
> *Gluten:*
> A plant protein found mostly in cereal grains.

Celiac disease is caused by intolerance to **gluten**. When a person with Celiac disease eats foods containing gluten, their immune system responds by attacking the substance within their small intestine. The collateral damage caused by the immune system can disrupt the intestine's ability to absorb nutrients, which causes afflicted individuals to become malnourished regardless of how much or how often they eat.

In my experience—if you're suffering from Celiac disease, you almost certainly have some form of stone-related liver/gallbladder malfunction. This is because the majority of toxins (including glutens) absorbed by the small intestine are eventually deposited in either the liver or gallbladder. It is not uncommon to expel 100 to 500 stones after performing a thorough liver/gallbladder cleanse!

What are the symptoms of Celiac Disease?

Many people with Celiac disease exhibit no symptoms at all. This is especially dangerous because these individuals are unaware of the damage occurring inside their bodies. When symptoms of CD surface, they can vary substantially from person to person.

SYMPTOMS OF CELIAC DISEASE MAY INCLUDE:

- Abdominal pain
- Bloating
- Diarrhea
- Excess gas
- Joint pain
- Menstrual problems
- Mouth sores
- Muscle cramps

- Fatigue
- Fertility problems
- Osteoporosis
- Tooth discoloration
- Skin irritation
- Tingling in the legs
- Seizures
- Weight changes

The damage caused to the small intestine, combined with poor nutrient absorption, can also place people with Celiac disease at an increased risk for developing colon cancer.

Who is at risk for developing Celiac disease?

Research on Celiac disease is scarce compared to other types of bowel disease, but it has been observed that Caucasian people (particularly those of European descent) are at higher risk (slightly less than 1 in 100) to develop the illness. Celiac disease is one of the most common genetic diseases in Western societies, affecting many "... healthy, average Americans", many of whom remain undiagnosed and are asymptomatic.[20] In many regions of Europe, it affects one out of 250 to 300 people. Celiac disease is diagnosed among African or Asian peoples at a lower rate of incidence (less than 1 in 200).[21]

Until recently, the incidence of CD appeared to be much lower in the U.S., but recent studies suggest it is nearly equal to that of European nations. Celiac disease may be one of the most common yet astonishingly under-diagnosed digestive illnesses!

How Does Regular Colon Cleansing Help Prevent Celiac Disease?

- Eliminates built up toxins in the bowel and keeps the intestinal walls clean

- Helps relieve pressure on the liver and gallbladder to reduce the number of stones formed
- Strengthens the intestinal walls to prevent leakage of toxins back into the liver
- Decreases transit time to reduce exposure of the bowel lining to wheat gluten

DOCTOR'S NOTE:
The most straightforward method of dealing with Celiac disease is to completely remove gluten from your diet. A large percentage of people also appear to get relief from Celiac disease by regularly performing colon, liver, gallbladder, parasite, and heavy metal cleanses to help remove impurities.

Inflammatory Bowel Disease: What Is It?

Inflammatory Bowel Disease (IBD) is one name for two very similar diseases, both of which cause destructive swelling and inflammation in the intestinal tract. The two conditions, Crohn's disease and Ulcerative Colitis, are characterized by nearly identical symptoms—this makes it difficult for even trained professionals to distinguish between them. Nearly one and a half million people in the United States alone suffer from one of these two diseases.[22]

Both of these diseases can produce especially gruesome effects in young children because one of the hallmark symptoms is persistent, bloody diarrhea. Loss of blood can quickly lead to anemia, malnourishment, and ultimately even stunted development of a growing mind and body. Moreover, witnessing blood in their child's stool can obviously cause a great deal of concern for any parent.

Crohn's Disease: Crohn's disease causes severe inflammation and swelling deep within the lining of the digestive tract. The swelling can be so painful that it forces the intestines to expel waste prematurely in the form of loose stool or diarrhea.

While Crohn's most commonly affects the intestines, it can also affect other portions of the digestive tract such as the mouth and stomach. In some cases, multiple sections of the digestive tract can be inflamed while the areas between them remain perfectly healthy.

What are the symptoms of Crohn's disease?

The two most widely reported symptoms of Crohn's disease are diarrhea and abdominal pain along the right side. Other symptoms of Crohn's disease may include weight loss, arthritis, skin problems, fever, and rectal bleeding (chronic bleeding can lead to anemia).

Crohn's disease is arguably the more severe of the two forms of IBD. Up to 75 percent of the people who suffer from Crohn's are advised to undergo surgery at least once, however "…Crohn's cannot be cured with surgery. Even if the diseased portion of the intestine is removed, the inflammation can reappear in a previously unaffected portion of the intestine."[23]

In fact, it's not uncommon for patients to undergo multiple rounds of surgery to remove damaged sections of their intestines in an effort to alleviate the symptoms of the disease. With regular colon cleansing and the addition of soil-based Probiotics, surgery can be avoided and the intestinal lining can begin to repair itself.

Who is at risk for Crohn's disease?

Crohn's disease is most often diagnosed in people between the ages of 20 and 30. Individuals with relatives who suffer from some form of IBD also run a much greater risk of developing Crohn's disease. Approximately 20 percent of people coping with Crohn's disease have a close blood relative (most often a brother or sister) with Inflammatory Bowel Disease. Being of Jewish ancestry also appears to significantly increase risk, while being

African American decreases the risk for this condition.[24]

How Does Regular Colon Cleansing Help Prevent Crohn's Disease?

- Eliminates built up toxins and cleanses the intestinal walls
- May prevent and reduce the inflammation of intestinal tissue
- Strengthens the intestinal walls, reinforcing weak spots that could be susceptible to Crohn's disease
- Sets up a hospitable environment for the natural balance of Probiotic strains needed to help repair the intestinal lining
- Decreases transit time, which reduces exposure of the bowel lining to toxins
- Helps restore proper bowel function, preventing the possibility of multiple surgeries

Ulcerative Colitis: Ulcerative colitis causes inflammation in the lining of the colon and rectum. The symptoms are similar to those seen in patients suffering from Crohn's disease, but Ulcerative Colitis does not affect the small intestine, mouth, esophagus, and stomach. The main difference between the two conditions is the depth of inflammation in the intestinal wall.

In Crohn's, all layers of the digestive tissue are susceptible; but with Colitis, only the surface of the intestinal lining is affected. Colitis completely destroys portions of the lining and leaves behind open sores or ulcers. These ulcers continuously leak blood and toxic pus back into the digestive system, which can further inflame the bowel and lead to more ulcers. In many ways, UC is like a fire that constantly pours gasoline on itself.

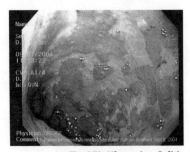

Fig. VII: Ulcerative Colitis viewed during Colonoscopy

What are the symptoms of Ulcerative Colitis?

Abdominal pain and bloody diarrhea are the most commonly experienced symptoms of UC. Sufferers of this condition have also reported fatigue, weight loss, and a change in appetite, skin lesions, and fever. Seemingly unrelated afflictions such as osteoporosis, arthritis, liver disease, and eye inflammation have been reported, but medical doctors still aren't sure exactly why. Drugs are usually prescribed to help control the symptoms of Colitis for as long as possible. Unfortunately these drugs aren't very effective, and about one-third of all patients diagnosed with this disease eventually have their colons removed. The majority of these surgeries are unnecessary and could be avoided with regular intestinal cleansing.

Who is at risk for Ulcerative Colitis?

People of Euro-Caucasian or Jewish ancestry (and ranging in age from childhood to young adulthood) possess a significantly higher risk for developing Colitis. As with Crohn's disease, being related to someone with Colitis also increases one's risk for being diagnosed with it. [25]

How Does Regular Colon Cleansing Help Prevent Ulcerative Colitis?

- Eliminates built up toxins and keeps the intestinal walls clean of toxic material
- Reduces the acid concentrations in the intestinal lining to prevent the development of ulcerated tissue
- Helps clean existing ulcerations and speeds up healing time of ulcerated tissue
- Decreases transit time, which reduces the constant irritation of the ulcers by hard, compacted fecal matter
- Helps restore proper mucous secretion, thereby lubricating the intestinal walls. This creates less irritation and friction around sites of ulceration

Colon Polyps: What Are They?

Colon polyps are small growths of tissue, similar to a large mole or wart that develops along the internal lining of the colon. Like regular moles on the skin, small polyps aren't usually dangerous. However, since some larger polyps can eventually develop into cancer, doctors routinely remove polyps of any size to be on the safe side. While most diverticular polyps will not develop into colon cancer, most internal colon polyps will.

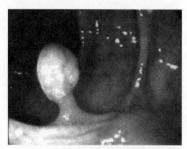

Fig. VIII: Colon Polyp viewed during Colonoscopy

What are the symptoms of Colon Polyps?

Typically, people with colon polyps don't notice any symptoms. Polyps can be very sneaky though, and many people discover they have them during a routine colonoscopy or sigmoidoscopy. It's not uncommon for people with polyps to experience symptoms such as constipation, diarrhea, and blood in the stool.

Who is at risk for getting Colon Polyps?

Your chances of developing polyps increase if ...

- You're over 40
- You've previously had polyps
- A relative or family member has had polyps
- A relative or family member has had colorectal cancer
- You consume high fat and fried foods
- You smoke tobacco or drink alcohol
- You don't exercise on a regular basis (2 to 3 times weekly)
- You are 15 or more pounds overweight
- You do not cleanse your liver, gallbladder, and intestinal tract on a regular basis

What treatment options are available for Colon Polyps?

The most common method for removing polyps is with a colonoscope during a colonoscopy. The polyps are then tested for malignancy. Once again, this addresses only the symptom and not the true cause. If polyps were there before, what is to say they will not just grow back? In the majority of cases, polyps do grow back. Keeping up with a healthy diet and exercise routine and avoiding as many colon toxins as possible is an excellent way to reduce your chances of developing polyps. I also recommend regular cleansing of the colon to help keep the intestinal lining free of toxic compaction that could lead to polyps.

How Does Regular Colon Cleansing Help Prevent Colon Polyps?

- Eliminates built up toxins and cleanses the intestinal walls of toxic material, reducing the chances of polyps developing
- Decreases transit time, which minimizes the constant irritation to the intestinal lining
- Reduces the size of polyps, which reduces their risk of developing into colon cancer
- Helps eliminate Candida and fungi suspected of initiating polyp growth

Colon Cancer: What Is It?

Colon cancer (or colorectal cancer) is one of the most common cancers in the United States and is spreading around the world at an alarming rate. Colorectal cancer is the third most common type of cancer [26] and approximately half of all cases result in death![27] That's a pretty scary statistic when you know practically all these cases could have been prevented.

Colon cancer normally develops when benign colon polyps become cancerous and damage the delicate intestinal tissue. My personal belief is that all cancers of the body develop from toxic overload in the liver and intestines, coupled with negative emotional stressors.

Illustration of Consecutive Stages of Colon Cancer

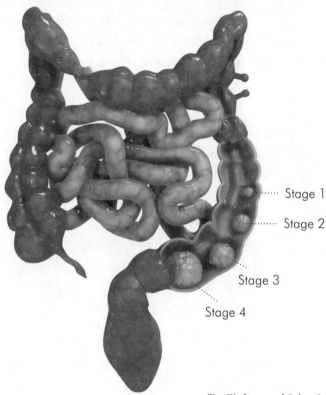

Fig. IX: Stages of Colon Cancer

What are the symptoms of Colon Cancer?

Remember that polyps often go undetected since most people present very few or no symptoms. It's scary, but the same is true for colon cancer that's caused by cancerous polyps. As the polyps slowly develop into cancer, many individuals experience no discomfort or other symptoms. However, some people experience bloody stools, abdominal pain, alternating bouts of diarrhea and constipation, weight loss, changes in appetite, anemia, fatigue, or pale complexion.

Who is at risk for Colon Cancer?

Everyone! Factors that may elevate your risk for developing colon cancer include: having polyps or inflammatory bowel disease, pre-existing cancer in another part of the body (particularly the breast), and having relatives with a history of colorectal cancer. A significant rise in the risk of colon cancer occurs for both males and females after age 35.[28] It's estimated 1 in 26 women (compared to 1 in 27 men), will suffer from the disease at some point in their life.[29] The biggest risk factor however is the amount of daily toxins to which you expose yourself.

Remember the Toxic Threshold mentioned in Chapter 2? Reducing these daily toxins from your environment is the easiest way to help prevent the development of colon cancer. People who are diagnosed in the early stages of the disease are much more likely to recover. Late detection of malignant polyps is one of the main reasons colorectal cancer accounts for an estimated 1 out of every 10 cancer-related deaths in the United States.[30]

How Does Regular Colon Cleansing Help Prevent Colon Cancer?

- Eliminates built-up toxins and rids the intestinal walls of toxic material, thereby reducing the chances of polyps becoming malignant
- Decreases the size of polyps, which reduces the risk of developing colon cancer
- Helps balance intestinal pH levels, reducing the acidic environment that promotes cancer development
- Prevents chronic fermentation in the bowels, reducing the levels of glucose. Glucose (especially refined sugar) is the main source of food for cancerous tissue growth

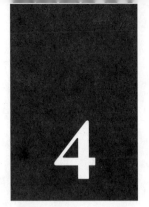

CHAPTER FOUR

HOW HEALTHY IS YOUR COLON?

It's not a common topic of conversation, so most of us don't give much thought to colon health or pay close attention to our bowel patterns. But, if you're serious about restoring and maintaining your health, you have to start paying more attention to your colon by monitoring your bowel movements. As odd as it may sound, you have to investigate what you eliminate!

It's hard to know exactly what's "normal". After all, everyone's body operates a little differently, and we're each exposed to different environments, diets, living conditions, and lifestyles. Nonetheless, you can take advantage of some general indicators to check for normal, healthy bowel movements.

Stools should typically be soft and easy to pass. If you experience bloating, gas, bad breath, skin blemishes, hard or pellet-like stools, less than 3 bowel movements daily, or you have to strain during bowel movements even once or twice a week, there's a good chance you're colon is not healthy. Ideally, stools should be brown or golden brown, shaped like sausage, and resemble peanut butter in overall texture.

Unfortunately, many of us consistently experience abnormal bowel movements without realizing it. Constipation and diarrhea have become two of the most common conditions afflicting practically everyone in the world. These disorders have become so normal, in fact, that we don't see them for what they really are—a cry for help from our colons!

For healthcare professionals to better diagnose these conditions and others affecting the bowels, a standardized tool was created to evaluate the size, shape, and consistency of stool.

The Bristol Stool Scale

Originally developed in 1997 by a small team of gastroenterologists at the University of Bristol in the United Kingdom, the Bristol Stool Scale was designed to be a general measurement system for healthcare professionals to evaluate stool consistency and form.[31] Simply put, this scale is a medical tool for classifying bowel movements (as they appear in toilet water) into seven distinct categories. A direct correlation exists between the form of the stool and the amount of time it has spent in the colon (due to factors such as hydration, constipation or lack thereof, diet, etc.).

You don't have to be a digestive health expert to benefit from using the Bristol Stool Scale. It can easily be used at home to analyze everyday bowel movements. The scale can also be a useful tool for noting sudden changes in your digestive habits and determining if your colon is functioning as it should.

The Bristol Stool Chart

TYPE 1  SEPARATE HARD LUMPS, LIKE NUTS (HARD TO PASS)

TYPE 2 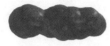 SAUSAGE-SHAPED BUT LUMPY

TYPE 3 (NORMAL)  LIKE A SAUSAGE BUT WITH CRACKS ON ITS SURFACE

TYPE 4 (NORMAL)  LIKE A SAUSAGE OR SNAKE, SMOOTH AND SOFT

TYPE 5  SOFT BLOBS WITH CLEAR-CUT EDGES (PASSED EASILY)

TYPE 6 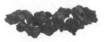 FLUFFY PIECES WITH RAGGED EDGES, A MUSHY STOOL

TYPE 7  WATERY, NO SOLID PIECES, ENTIRELY LIQUID

DR. GROUP HAS ADDED THIS CATEGORY TO THE ORIGINAL 7.

TYPE 8 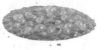 FOUL-SMELLING, MUCUS-LIKE WITH BUBBLES (SPRAYED OUT)

Fig. X

Analyzing Your Stool[32]

Type 1: Stools appear in separate, hard lumps, similar to nuts. Type 1 stools have spent the longest amount of time in the colon and are generally difficult to pass. Type 1 stools are a sure sign that you're constipated, full of toxins, and in need of regular intestinal cleansing. These are the most common stools among individuals.

Type 2: Stools are sausage-like in appearance but lumpy. These stools also indicate you are constipated, toxic, and need regular intestinal cleansing.

Type 3 (Normal): Stools come out similar to a sausage but with cracks in the surface. Type 3 stools are considered normal.

Type 4 (Normal): Stools are smooth and soft in the form of a sausage or snake. Type 4 stools are also considered normal.

Type 5: Stools form soft blobs with clear-cut edges that are easily passed through the digestive system. Type 5 stools are classified as soft diarrhea and are a possible risk for bowel disease. These stools also indicate you are toxic and need regular intestinal cleansing.

Type 6: Stools have fluffy pieces with ragged edges. These are considered mushy stools, and indicate diarrhea. These stools also indicate that you are toxic and need regular intestinal cleansing.

Type 7: Stool is mostly liquid with no solid pieces. This type of stool has spent the least amount of time in the colon. This indicates severe diarrhea due to cholera or a bacterial or viral infection. See a doctor as soon as possible.

The following is my addition and not part of the original Bristol Stool Scale.

Type 8: Stool has foul odor and is mucous-like with bubbles (sprayed out). This indicates excessive intake of alcohol and/or recreational drugs. Please seek help for removing alcohol or drugs from your life.

Note: *If you are experiencing Type 1, 2, 5, 6, 7, or 8 stools for longer than 1 month, I recommend you perform* The Oxygen Colon Cleanse *in Chapter 5, followed by 3 consecutive Liver/Gallbladder Cleanses (see Chapter 12). Start by eliminating toxins from your diet and environment. You may also want to see your healthcare provider to determine the root cause of your problem.*

> **DEFINITION**
>
> *Protein:*
> large organic compounds made of amino acids. Animal proteins are not easily digestible by humans, especially if the stomach does not produce enough digestive fluids.

Stools with a really foul odor may result from an imbalance of intestinal bacteria or from consuming too much animal **protein.** A rancid foul-smelling odor lurking for more than 3 to 5 minutes in the bathroom after evacuation is a definite sign you need to cleanse your colon. Your body is trying to get your attention with that odor—something is wrong inside of you! The longer you ignore this, the more damage you will have. Your colon is practically screaming at you to change your dietary habits! Most people are not taught these critical signs and therefore do not listen to their bodies.

PLEASE PAY ATTENTION TO THE SIGNS YOUR BODY GIVES YOU!

According to current medical science, Types 3 and 4 stools (***if passed once every three days***) qualify as "normal." I strongly disagree with this as I firmly believe you should have at least two Type 3 or 4 bowel movements every single day.

In general, constipated people produce stools that are categorized as either Type 1 or Type 2. Research indicates over 60 million people live with the daily discomfort of passing unhealthy bowel movements.[33]

People suffering from diarrhea pass Type 5, 6, or 7 stools on an uncomfortably frequent basis. Every year, over 21 million Americans experience diarrhea at some point.[34]

Should I Look for Anything Else in My Stool?

Yes! **Mucous** in the stool can be a symptom of digestive problems or

> **DEFINITION**
>
> **Mucous:**
> a slippery or slimy secretion produced by any number of bodily membranes.

it can be a result of a successful colon cleansing. Knowing the difference between the two is largely dependent upon the circumstances. Either way, it's important to be able to recognize mucous in your stool.

Mucous can also be caused by eating unhealthy foods, or foods to which you may be allergic such as dairy products. With food allergens, the intestinal wall produces extra mucous to protect itself. Since most people follow unhealthy diets, it's not unusual for the digestive system to produce excess mucous.

How Do I Identify Mucous in My Stool?

Mucous is generally pretty easy to identify. In all cases, mucous has a slimy consistency, but it can be white, yellow, or clear in color. Mucous may cover the entire surface of a bowel movement or may appear as small particles that are sometimes mistaken for worms.

Seeing mucous in your stool isn't necessarily a sign of a problem. In fact, the large intestine naturally produces some protective mucous to trap foreign particles and move waste through the colon. Since mucous serves to protect your digestive system, it's not unusual to find increased amounts of mucous when you're suffering from constipation or diarrhea.

When Does the Presence of Mucous Indicate Trouble?

If you experience mucous only occasionally, you shouldn't be too concerned about it. If you produce mucous for more than a few weeks or if it's accompanied by a foul smell or bleeding, you should consult with a healthcare professional as soon as possible. These additional symptoms may indicate a serious health problem.

Mucous-Covered Stools could be a warning sign for:

Ulcerative Colitis, Irritable Bowel Syndrome, Infection, or Bowel Obstruction.

What Do Colored Stools Indicate?

> **DEFINITION**
>
> **Biliary system:** the organs and duct system that create, carry, store and release bile into the small intestine.

Green Stool: Green bowel movements can be caused by several factors, mostly related to dietary issues. In most cases, green stools are harmless but they can indicate a digestive disorder. If you can attribute a green bowel movement to something you've eaten recently, it's not a cause for concern. If you consistently produce green bowel movements, further investigation with your healthcare professional may be necessary.

Bile is also green in color and is secreted by the liver directly into the small intestine or stored in the gallbladder. Bile is released to break down fats. As normal stool passes from the small intestine to the colon, it changes from green to yellow to brown. When transit time is increased due to an underlying condition, your bowel movements can take on a green color. It is also normal for breast-fed infants to have green looking stools due to the Colostrum in breastmilk.

Some Common Causes of Green Stool

- Food passing through the digestive system too quickly (due to food poisoning, food allergies, or a stomach virus)
- Vitamins or supplements with large amounts of iron
- Eating an excessive amount of sugar
- Consuming too many green, leafy vegetables and not enough grains
- Taking algae or chlorophyll supplements
- Performing a liver/gallbladder cleanse (due to purged toxins)

White Stool: White stool can indicate trouble with the kidneys or **biliary system** since bile is responsible for creating the colors commonly seen in waste matter. If a problem exists with these systems, the bile may not be formulated correctly and a white bowel movement can occur. If you have a bowel movement that is solid white all the way through, it's important to seek immediate medical attention from a physician specializing in digestive disorders!

If your body digests food too quickly, you might also experience a white bowel movement. In this case, the white color is due to mucous, not bile. If waste passes through your body too fast, the mucous produced by your colon may not be digested before the stool is eliminated.

Although this may not sound especially pleasant, you can determine the cause of your white bowel movement by soaking the stool in water. If it is just a mucous-covered stool, the white mucous should disintegrate, leaving behind normal looking waste matter. White stools caused by problems with bile production, however, will remain white.

Having a small amount of mucous in your stool is considered normal since your digestive system naturally produces it for efficient waste removal. Large amounts of mucous, on the other hand, are not normal and may require further action.

Yellow Stool: Yellow stool often indicates a condition know as "pale stool" in which the stool is pale or yellow in color. Unless (for some strange reason) you ingested massive amounts of food coloring, yellow stool is not normal. If your stool is pale or yellow, your large intestine, liver, small intestine, or stomach may be affected by a serious condition or disease.

Additional Features of Unhealthy Stool

If bowel movements are:	It may be due to...
Dark black and sticky (Seek immediate medical attention!)	Blood in the upper portion of the digestive tract
Very dark brown	Recent red wine consumption, an excess of salt, or lack of vegetable intake
Beet red	Eating red foods
Super thin, resembling a ribbon	Polyp development in the colon
Greasy looking	Insufficient absorption of nutrients

Take the Colon Health Self-Test

It's important to really know your body before a treatment plan can begin. The following test can provide you with valuable information about the health of your colon as well as your risk of developing serious intestinal problems.

Simply answer Yes or No to the list of questions. *Remember—be honest!* If you find some of the questions difficult to answer off the top of your head, you may first want to keep a journal of your bowel habits and general health for a week or so.

Base your answers on the last 30 days.

1) Do you run out of energy in the afternoon?
2) Do you suffer from occasional headaches? (1 to 2 per week?)
3) Are you having less than 2 or 3 normal bowel movements daily?
4) Do you have problems concentrating from time to time?
5) Do you experience gas or bloating 1 or more times weekly?
6) Do you get irritable from time to time?
7) Do you have difficulty getting a good night's rest?
8) Do you have muscle aches and/or stiffness?
9) Do you eat red meat more than 2 times per week?
10) Do you eat fried foods more than twice per week?
11) Do you drink less than ½ gallon of purified water daily?

12) Do you have problems controlling your weight?

13) Do you exercise less than 3 times weekly?

14) Do you suffer from allergies or sinus problems?

15) Do you have bad breath or body odor?

16) Are you unhappy with your current health?

17) Are you currently suffering from any health problems?

18) Do you have hemorrhoids?

19) Is your skin dry, broken, spotted, or blemished in any way?

20) Do you have occasional abdominal pain?

21) Do you have to strain to have a bowel movement?

22) Do your bowel movements have a foul odor?

23) Do you have hard, small, or dry stools 1 to 2 times weekly?

24) Do you notice bright red blood on the toilet paper one or more times per month?

25) Do you have painful bowel movements?

26) Do you use a microwave to cook more than 2 meals per week?

27) Do you drink coffee, soft drinks, alcohol, or milk more than 2 times per week?

28) Are you currently taking any prescription medications?

If you answered "Yes" to 8 or more questions, your bowel is not functioning properly and you have likely exceeded your daily Toxic Threshold. Now that you've assessed the current health of your colon, you're ready to learn more about the benefits of cleansing, plus how **The Oxygen Colon Cleanse** can jumpstart your health and help you maintain an efficient digestive tract.

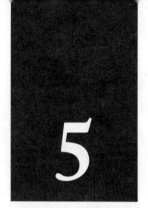

CHAPTER FIVE

THE OXYGEN COLON CLEANSE

To review, so far you've learned about the different types of colon disease and you now know that acquired disease starts in the intestinal tract. Hopefully, by this point, you also know how healthy or unhealthy your colon is. This chapter will cover the most effective ways to cleanse your entire intestinal tract from beginning to end. I will finish the chapter with other methods for cleansing and maintaining general intestinal health. I must state again that prevention is the best way to maintain maximum health. Part II- How to Live in a Green, Toxin Free Environment *explains in detail* how toxins in your living environment affect you on a daily basis and how to reduce your Toxic Threshold by eliminating these toxins once and for all.

If you're like most of the people I talk to about colon cleansing, you're probably overwhelmed by the sheer variety of cleansing options out there. The good news is—more and more people seem to be catching on to the importance of regular intestinal cleansing. Unfortunately, it also seems that many supplement companies are just out to make a quick buck from the growing digestive health movement.

The majority of the products you find in drugstores, supermarkets, wholesale clubs, television, and on the Internet are nothing more than cheaply made concoctions that may cause further problems. If these products are good for anything at all, it's cleaning out your wallet.

Before I continue, I must say CONGRATULATIONS to YOU on reading this book and making the commitment to transform your health! In this chapter, you're going to discover how to avoid the years of misery and frustration afflicting millions of Americans every day because they don't have access to the special information within this book.

Now, I invite you to relax, close your eyes, and picture in your mind a day without bothersome bloating and gas, fatigue, headaches, and any other symptoms you may be experiencing. A day where you feel self-confident, happy, full of life, and worry-free.

Can you imagine that day? What favorite activity are you doing? How healthy and happy do you feel? With whom are you spending that time? Isn't a moment like that what life is all about?

Did you know you can transform that fantasy into your reality? How would you like to finally get rid of your negative health concerns and live in a normal, healthy body? No more stress, no more irritation, no more feeling sluggish—you can live with happiness, joy, and peace.

I've spent years helping people like you discover the truth about their health problems and teaching them how to feel healthy again quickly, easily, and naturally (without any drugs, surgery, or toxic side effects)!

I wrote this book because, frankly, I became sick of seeing people feeling lousy and insecure with themselves or experiencing a lifetime of misery because no one would reveal to them the secret to health!

In fact, I practice and teach skills solely on cleansing the body. Nothing is more pleasing than helping people just like you to finally live life on their terms again!

However, I feel I have to warn you—it's in your best interest to act right now; if you procrastinate on your health, your body might deteriorate to the point where I can no longer help you. Either way, I wish you good luck and a bright future in the light of excellent health!

"Keeping the colon clean is that which is necessary for every well-balanced body; hence should be a part of the experience for each entity." [35]

-Edgar Cayce

I developed the following cleanse protocol for people wanting a deep, thorough cleansing of their entire intestinal tract and colon. I recommend performing the 6-Day Oxygen Colon Cleanse at least three to four times per year and following up with regular maintenance cleansing 2 or 3 times weekly.

The 6-Day Oxygen Colon Cleanse

This advanced cleanse requires using an oxygen-based cleanser because I believe they are the safest and most effective. If you would like to jump-start the cleansing process, you may also want to receive a colon hydrotherapy session first.

Supplies Needed for the 6-Day Oxygen Colon Cleanse:

1. 6 gallons of distilled water
2. 8 ounces of organic, raw, non-pasteurized Apple Cider Vinegar (ACV)
3. 3 organic lemons (If you cannot find organic or locally grown then use fresh lemons from your supermarket)
4. 1 bottle of Oxy-Powder® or another high-quality oxygen-based intestinal cleanser
5. 1 Bottle of Latero-Flora® or another excellent Probiotic formula
6. Fresh fruit–Preferably organic or locally grown
7. 16 ounces of Organic Whole Leaf Cold Pressed Aloe Vera Juice. (I recommend R PUR Aloe International® 18X Concentrate. See also "Aloe Vera" in the *Resources* section).

Note: If you purchase aloe juice from your local health food store, make sure it's the highest quality available (without any added sugars and preferably organic).

Making the Intestinal Cleanser

Try to drink 1 gallon of the Intestinal Cleanser every day during the 6-Day Cleanse. It is best to keep your Intestinal Cleanser refrigerated throughout the day. If you are not able to finish the gallon by the end of the day, discard the rest and start fresh the following day. Do your best to finish 1 gallon per day.

Daily Instructions:

1. Start with 1 gallon of distilled water
2. Pour out 4 ounces of the distilled water
3. Add 2 tablespoons of organic Apple Cider Vinegar (Available at most grocery stores or health food stores.) Shake the ACV well before adding
4. Add 2 ounces of R PUR Aloe International® 18X Concentrate or

organic Aloe juice from your local health food store

5. Add the juice of ½ lemon
6. Mix well and keep refrigerated

Why is Organic Apple Cider Vinegar in the Intestinal Cleanser?

Apple Cider Vinegar may be one of nature's most potent detoxifiers against a variety of negative health conditions. Created through the fermentation of raw apples within wooden barrels, vinegar from apple cider is extremely acidic (with a **pH** around 2.8) and this may be the key factor of its amazing curative powers.

> **DEFINITION**
>
> *pH:*
> stands for potential Hydrogen and is a measure of acidity and alkalinity.
>
> *Mother:*
> essentially, a structure of protein filaments clinging together that resembles a spider's web.

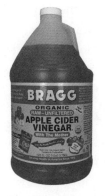

Bragg™ Organic ACV

The greater the purity of the apples utilized in the fermentation process, the greater the health benefits and detoxifying power for you. Only fresh organically grown apples (that have not been treated with pesticides and chemical fertilizers or undergone genetic modification) are used.

Organic Apple Cider Vinegar contains fibrous pectin and the "mother" or "the veil of the mother." The **mother** is usually visible floating in the vinegar when it's held up to the light. You'll see a minute cloudiness within the vinegar appearing like tiny grains or strands. These particles add fiber to the ACV and ensure you receive the most beneficial components of the original apples—essential vitamins, minerals, enzymes, and amino acids. Nearly a hundred different health-promoting substances have been identified in organic Apple Cider Vinegar.

Caution: Most non-organic brands of ACV undergo pasteurization (boiled at high heat to remove bacteria), and filtration, leaving you with a form so refined that it's nutritionally worthless.

ACV is arguably one of the best all-around detoxifiers for your body's intestinal tract and organs. Once the body is detoxified, it can begin the process of self-healing from an array of diseases and ailments. This is why it's so important to use only organic Apple Cider Vinegar—it's the only way to obtain all the life-promoting enzymes and vitamins needed for proper intestinal detoxification. ACV also inhibits the growth of harmful yeast, germs, fungi, and bacteria in the intestinal tract, thereby increasing the absorption and utilization of vital nutrients.

High quality sources of Organic Apple Cider Vinegar include: Solana Gold™ Virtues of Vinegar Organic ACV[36], Bragg™ Organic ACV[37], and Spectrum™ Organic ACV[38].

Why is Aloe Vera Juice in the Intestinal Cleanser?

The structural composition of an Aloe Vera plant includes the very building blocks of life: essential vitamins and minerals, proteins, polysaccharides, enzymes, and amino acids. Therefore, the Aloe plant's internal makeup closely relates to human biochemistry and its juice provides many positive health benefits.

Aloe Vera possesses multiple natural qualities for healing and detoxifying the body. When taken internally, Aloe aids the bowel in flushing out accumulated waste and toxic debris. Aloe Vera can help ease a variety of constipation symptoms, improve regularity in bowel movements, and keep the colon clean.

Aloe Vera Juice (from the whole leaf) is helpful in alleviating a number of digestive disorders such as:

- Acid indigestion
- Bloating and gas
- Candida
- Colitis
- Constipation
- Diarrhea
- Hemorrhoids
- Irritable Bowel Syndrome
- Poor appetite

- Sluggish bile production
- Ulcers

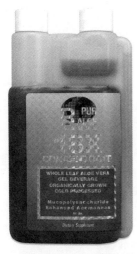

R PUR Aloe International®

Aloe Vera contains a large number of mucopolysacchrides (basic sugars) which are found in every cell in the body. As mentioned, Aloe contains essential compounds that enhance nutrient absorption and overall digestive function. With more than 200 valuable substances, Aloe Vera provides many other health benefits.

Aloe Vera's tissue regeneration properties work towards rebuilding tissue of the stomach and intestinal tract. Such tissue can become damaged through disease or even extended bouts of constipation, and researchers have found that Aloe Vera stimulates fibroblasts into constructing new tissue. Aloe polysaccharides improve immune system strength and are very effective at eliminating toxin-filled waste by boosting the body's natural detoxification processes.

In any event, an important fact must be remembered—Aloe Vera presents no known side effects and is quite safe. Throughout history, the Aloe Vera plant has been universally regarded as nature's gift for treating burns, skin conditions, and digestive difficulties.

I recommend R PUR Aloe International® because they have mastered the whole leaf processing method. It is prepared by a new and revolutionary whole leaf cold process to ensure maximum efficacy and it exceeds all International Standards for Aloe Processing (ISAP).

Traditional methods of refining the Aloe Vera plant involve a hand filleting process to remove the gel from the leaf. The leaf is then discarded. Ironically, the largest concentration of the active ingredients, polysaccharides, and mucopolysacchride (Acemannan), are found just beneath the outer surface of the leaf (the rind), which can be bitter, indigestible, possibly abrasive, and difficult to refine.

The new whole leaf process employed in the making of the Aloe Vera 18X Concentrate allows the cellulose to be dissolved so the aloin and aloe emodin are removed. The cold process results in a product rich in polysaccharides including mucopolysaccharides (MPS). For these reasons, I personally use this product.

Why is Lemon Juice in the Intestinal Cleanser?

Drinking freshly squeezed lemon juice while cleansing provides an incredible nutrient boost for your colon. Due to the amazing digestive properties of lemons, the juice maximizes The 6-Day Oxygen Colon Cleanse by providing the following benefits:

- It removes impurities from the intestinal tract and body
- Its antiseptic properties reduce the presence of harmful bacteria within the bowel
- Helps alleviate symptoms of heartburn, excess gas, and bloating
- Helps the bowels eliminate waste more efficiently, reducing possible diarrhea or constipation
- Stimulates the liver for enhanced enzyme production
- Helps create an alkaline condition within the body

Lemons are one of the only "anionic" foods, meaning they possess a greater number of negative ions than positive ones. Most of the fluids produced by the digestive system (such as bile, stomach acid, and saliva) are also anionic, so lemon juice is quite compatible with your digestive system.

To receive the natural healing properties present in lemons, it's important to use whole, fresh, organic lemons. Lemons from a grocery store are usually not as "pure" as you might believe due to over-processing, early picking, pesticide spraying, or being grown in nutrient-depleted soil.

Using fresh squeezed, organic lemon juice helps you eliminate more toxins on a daily basis. The more toxins you can flush out of your system, the more your colon will be receptive to your cleansing efforts.

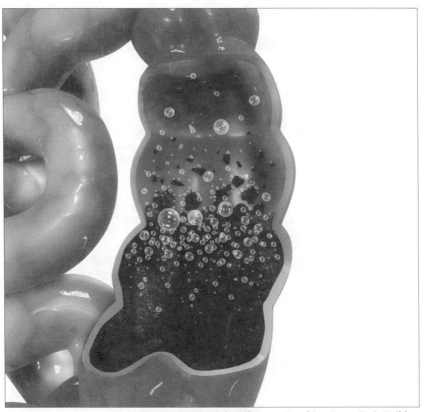

Fig. XI: Oxygen Colon Cleanser Breaking Down Toxic Buildup

Why Are Oxygen-Based Colon Cleansers Used?

As far as I'm concerned, the most effective way to cleanse the entire intestinal tract and colon is with an oxygen-based cleanser.

This type of cleanser uses a controlled reaction to release pure singlet oxygen straight into the bowels. What exactly is singlet oxygen? Well, it might sound like something technical and complicated, but it's really just a single, un-bonded oxygen atom (O_1). The air you breathe is actually O_2, or 2 oxygen molecules bonded together.

Most oxygen-based cleansers use specialized forms of ozonated magnesium oxides to break down the solid toxic mass into a liquid or gas, so it is easily passed from the body. Basically, oxygen "singlet" atoms are bonded to a magnesium compound. The hydrochloric acid in your

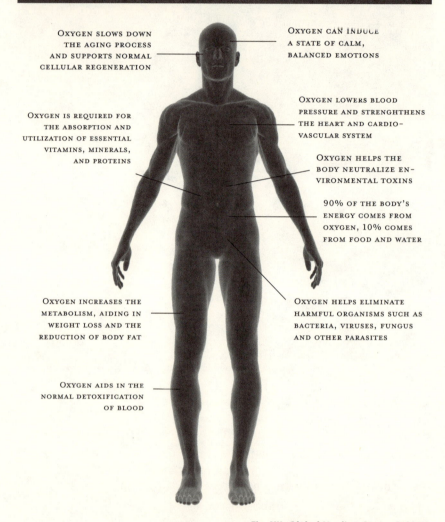

Fig. XII: Global Healing Center © 2007

stomach (along with the organic lemon juice and other acids in your bowel) releases these bonds, thus allowing oxygen to escape into the intestines.

Oxygen is a lively element, and if you're using a high quality oxygen cleanser, it will pump enough oxygen into your bowels to literally burrow through the toxic sludge and contaminated mucous caked on the sides of your intestines. The vital oxygen provided by these cleansers helps to purge garbage from the colon and it also serves as an excellent remedy for constipation and IBS as proven in human clinical trials.

As the years of waste melt away, the intestinal lining hidden beneath is revealed. In most cases, this lining is littered with microscopic holes due to years of abuse. In a toxic colon, these holes allow toxins to enter the bloodstream. After cleansing the colon, however, these same holes present a perfect opportunity for oxygen to work its way into the bloodstream where it can help detoxify the entire body.

I should point out not all oxygen-based intestinal cleansers are created equally. As with any health product, it's important to conduct your own research before you start experimenting with your body. Many so-called oxygen cleansers simply don't release enough oxygen to do any good.

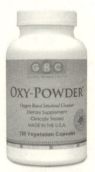

Oxy-Powder® Oxygen Intestinal Cleanser

In independent laboratory tests, only two oxygen-based cleansing products have been measured as releasing the amounts of oxygen needed to thoroughly cleanse the intestines. These two products are Homozon™[39] and Oxy-Powder®.[40]

Homozon™ has been around since the early 1900's and is considered to be the "grandfather" of all oxygen cleansers. In many ways, it's a product shrouded in mystery—its exact manufacturing process remains a secret to this day and there's even debate over who developed the original formula. Some say the famous inventor Nicola Tesla and Dr. Eugene Blass developed the process in a hotel room in Paris. While Homozon™ is an amazing product, it's not very widely marketed so it's difficult to find.

Okay, up until this point, I've avoided making any shameless plugs to promote my personal line of health supplements; but in this particular case, it would be irresponsible for me not to make an exception.

For years, I exclusively used Homozon™ and recommended it to my patients. Repeatedly, I was stunned by its effectiveness. I saw people's health make a complete turnaround, sometimes literally overnight. Of all the oxygen cleansers I researched, Homozon™ really stood out over the copycat oxygen cleansers.

Needless to say, I had (and still have) much respect for this product. But over the years, I began to notice some drawbacks and complaints from customers. First, the product was hard to get and we would have to wait 2 months or longer before receiving a very small shipment. Second, Homozon™ is a loose powder that has to be mixed with water and lemon juice. This concoction gives it a very peculiar and chalky taste. Many patients would not take this product as often as they should due to the taste, or they would gag while trying to swallow it!

I knew the world needed access to a product that was as safe and effective as Homozon™ but in an easy-to-take vegetarian capsule for continued use.

Years later (with the help of a world-renowned oxygen biochemist), Oxy-Powder® was born! By utilizing the advancements in technology made over the past 100 years, we generated a product proven to be more effective than any other oxygen-based colon cleanser in the world! With the addition of organic Germanium-132, we formulated a secret weapon for maintaining intestinal health via oxygen delivery. Germanium-132 can improve the health of arteries, lower blood pressure, help suppress some forms of cancer, inhibit the growth of fungi, and also enhance the body's utilization of oxygen.[41] This superior formulation is why I recommend Oxy-Powder® in my 6-Day Oxygen Colon Cleanse protocol.

Why is Latero-Flora™ or other Probiotics recommended during the 6-Day Oxygen Colon Cleanse?

An agriculturalist visiting a remote part of Iceland discovered rich tasting vegetables produced without chemicals. Returning to the U.S.A., the agriculturalist conducted a series of studies to determine the secret of the soil's growing power. The secret was a unique Probiotic strain of *Bacillus laterosporus* (B.O.D. STRAIN), a naturally occurring bacterium that was later incorporated into Latero-Flora™. In my many years of practice, I have tried numerous Probiotics. I recommend Latero-Flora™

because I have seen the most dramatic results with this product. Latero-Flora™ has demonstrated significant effectiveness in easing gastrointestinal symptoms and food sensitivities while enhancing digestive function. If you choose to use your own brand of Probiotics during the 6-Day Oxygen Colon Cleanse, or on a regular basis, research these supplements well and make sure you are using a very high quality product.

Just as the Earth holds an abundance of life forms (sometimes existing harmoniously, while struggling fitfully at other times), the human body likewise harbors a vast internal ecosystem consisting of thousands of billions of living microorganisms that co-exist in peace or in conflict.

This vast internal ecosystem (referred to by many researchers as "human intestinal flora") dramatically influences and even directs each person's state of health and well-being, including our physical and mental health and metabolism. Hundreds of distinct species of microorganisms inhabit the various regions of the complete digestive system (from the mouth through the intestinal tract). Their population (over 100 trillion) can actually exceed the number of cells in the entire body![42]

When functioning properly, this vast unseen world:

- Helps protect your body against harmful bacteria
- Helps maintain the function of the digestive system
- Maintains your body's vital chemical and hormone balance
- Performs a vast number of needed tasks for maintaining high energy levels and proper immune function

Transient microorganisms are especially worth noting. These "transients" include food-borne microorganisms and soil-borne microorganisms that make their way into the human digestive tract and, depending upon the characteristics of the organism involved, influence the overall health of the human system for good or ill.

Since they do not take up permanent residence in the gastrointestinal tract, transient microorganisms differ from resident microorganisms.

Transient Probiotics establish small colonies for brief periods of time before dying off or being flushed from the intestinal system via normal digestive processes or by peristaltic bowel action. However, in taking up temporary residence, they contribute to the overall function and condition of the digestive system. For example, the lives of some of the most important resident probiotics involved in human digestion and intestinal health depend on byproducts produced by the transient probiotics.

Therefore, in many cases, these two very different types of microorganisms nonetheless enjoy a complex symbiotic relationship that may dramatically influence the health and well being of your entire body. *Bacillus laterosporus* (B.O.D.™ strain) is one of the most rare and unique of the "friendly" transient microorganisms found in the human gastrointestinal tract. *Bacillus laterosporus* is a spore-bearing bacterium. This enables the encased spore to survive exposure to stomach acids. Thus, the *Bacillus laterosporus* B.O.D.™ will bloom and flourish in the colon and establish colonies that enhance your immune system and cleanse the colon of unwanted organisms such as Candida.

How does eating fresh fruit help?

During the 6-Day Oxygen Colon Cleanse, it's ideal to feed the body adequate amounts of fresh organic or locally grown fruit. It is best to eat only fruit during the 6-Day Cleanse. Not only does fruit supply the body with the right kind of energy to draw out unwanted substances, it also ensures the colon remains well hydrated so it's an ideal environment to support the cleansing and toxin elimination process. Fresh fruit supports the elimination process by providing water, oxygen, live fiber, pectin, and many vital nutrients.

Also, fruit is easy to carry with you wherever you go (even in your purse or briefcase), making it easy for you to perform the 6-Day Cleanse during work hours or other daily activities. Fruits provide you with the energy you will need during your cleansing regimen. Fruits also break down easily and prevent the body from expending too much energy. You should eat 5 times daily during the 6-Day Cleanse. This might sound difficult, but when you think about it, it really only takes about 2 minutes to peel and enjoy a banana or eat an apple or a bunch of grapes.

The fruits in the following chart have been specially chosen to assist you in the cleansing process. It is best to keep a little variety in the fruits you eat throughout the day and the week. If the fruits I recommend are not in season or you have a difficult time finding them, you can use apples or bananas (which are typically available year round) as a replacement.

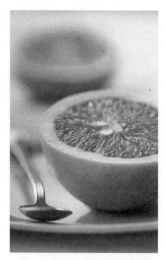

Example: I recommend eating grapefruit, white grapes, pineapple, or oranges for the breakfast and mid-afternoon meals. Although you could eat grapefruit for both meals, it is better if you eat a different selection of fruits at each meal.

The Oxygen Colon Cleanse Fruits		
Apples	Grapefruit	Strawberries
Avocado	Oranges	Tomatoes
Bananas	Papaya	Watermelon
Blackberries	Pineapples	White grapes
Blueberries	Raspberries	

NOTE: I'm sure you've heard this since childhood, but it really is essential to chew each bite of food 25 times before swallowing (or, in the case of fruit, until it has turned into a liquid). Proper digestion begins in the mouth with proper chewing! Chewing your food will help your body absorb vital nutrients better and faster and will help with the cleansing process. See *Chapter 6—The Colon Diet* for more details and tips on choosing healthful foods.

The 6-Day Oxygen Colon Cleanse

Days 1 to 6

UPON AWAKENING

1. Make your daily Intestinal Cleanser drink. Drink 20 ounces from the time you make your drink till the time you eat breakfast.
2. Repeat the following Affirmation 9 times: *I Am Clean and Healthy.*

BREAKFAST

1. Eat as much fruit as you can until you are full, but eat only 1 type of fruit!
2. Choose 1 of the following: grapefruit, white grapes, pineapple, oranges, or watermelon. If these are not in season substitute with apples or bananas.
3. After Breakfast and before your Mid-Morning Snack, consume another 20 ounces of the Intestinal Cleanser drink.
4. Repeat the following Affirmation 9 times: *I Am Clean and Healthy.*
5. Take 3 capsules of Latero-Flora™ or another high quality Probiotic supplement.

MID-MORNING SNACK (halfway between breakfast and lunch)

1. Eat as much fruit as you can until you are full. Only eat 1 type of fruit!
2. Choose one of the following: blackberries, raspberries, strawberries, or blueberries. If berries are not in season, replace them with apples or bananas.
3. After your Mid-Morning Snack and before your Lunch, consume another 20 ounces of the Intestinal Cleanser drink.
4. Repeat the following Affirmation 9 times: *I Am Clean and Healthy.*

LUNCH

1. Eat as much fruit as you can until you are full. Only eat 1 type of fruit!
2. Choose one of the following: apples, papaya, or bananas.
3. After Lunch and before your Mid-Afternoon Snack, consume another 20 ounces of the Intestinal Cleanser drink.
4. Repeat the following Affirmation 9 times: *I Am Clean and Healthy.*

MID-AFTERNOON SNACK (halfway between lunch and dinner):

1. Eat as much fruit as you can until you are full. Only eat 1 type of fruit!
2. Choose one of the following: grapefruit, white grapes, pineapple, or oranges
3. After your Mid-Afternoon Snack and before your Dinner, consume another 20 ounces of the Intestinal Cleanser drink.
4. Repeat the following Affirmation 9 times: *I Am Clean and Healthy.*

DINNER

1. Eat as much fruit as you can until you are full. Only eat 1 type of fruit!
2. Choose one of the following: avocados or tomatoes (tomatoes need to be vine ripened for best results). You may use fresh lime juice, natural sea salt (preferably Himalayan), cayenne or black pepper to season the avocado, or tomato if necessary. However, it is best to eat these vegetables raw.
3. After your dinner meal and before bedtime consume another 20 ounces of the Intestinal Cleanser drink.
4. Repeat the following Affirmation 9 times: *I Am Clean and Healthy.*

BEFORE BED

1. Repeat the following Affirmation 9 times: *I Am Clean and Healthy.*

2. Take 6 capsules of Oxy-Powder® or a good oxygen-based cleanser with the remaining 8 ounces of the Intestinal Cleanser drink. If you do not achieve 3 to 5 bowel movements the following day, increase your dosage by 2 capsules each night until you achieve 3 to 5 bowel movements the following day. Take this same dosage every night before going to bed for the remaining days of the 6-Day Oxygen Colon Cleanse. After you have completed the 6-Day Cleanse, take your maintenance dosage as needed.

Maintenance Dosing

To maintain a healthy intestinal tract, I recommend regular cleansing at least 2 times per week. Use the same dosage you used for your 6-Day Oxygen Colon Cleanse. This amount can be taken indefinitely without it becoming habit forming or harmful to your body. Taking a regular maintenance dose of an oxygen-based colon cleanser helps supply your entire body with beneficial oxygen and aids in the natural cleansing of your intestinal tract.

Once you have completed the cleanse, I recommend following the Colon Diet detailed in Chapter 6. After you read that chapter, you will be ready for the big task of slowly eliminating toxins from your environment. See Part 2 of this book.

6 TIPS to Maximize the Oxygen Colon Cleanse

1. Abdominal Massage

The abdomen is home to many of the most vital organs in the body. The abdominal cavity houses the stomach, gallbladder, pancreas, diaphragm, colon, small intestine, and the liver (collectively called the

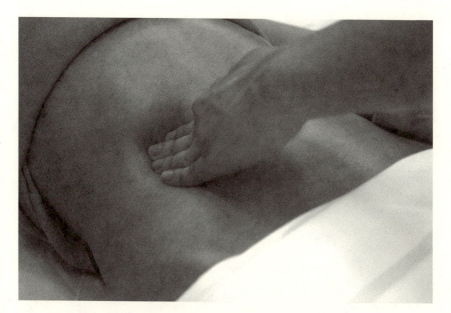

viscera). When something such as an illness or practicing a sedentary lifestyle weakens the digestive system, the abdomen can suffer. Abdominal massage is a method for keeping the internal muscles strong and it has been used by numerous cultures around the world for promoting overall health. Abdominal massage requires no prescription or special equipment plus you can perform it upon yourself as well as your friends, significant other, spouse, or children.

Some of the key benefits of abdominal massage include:

- Blood flow is increased within the abdominal cavity which, in turn, delivers more life-sustaining oxygen to the vital organs
- Helps remove toxins by stimulating internal detoxification processes
- Built up fecal matter is dislodged from the walls of the intestinal tract
- Provides basic comfort and soothing heat through touch therapy
- Aligns the pelvic bone and uterus in females to their proper positions
- Relieves tension and relaxes the muscles surrounding the colon, promoting a healthier digestive system
- Releases unprocessed emotional charges (tension)

Abdominal massage is highly recommended for anyone trying to detoxify their body. Practicing abdominal massage can greatly enhance the cleansing procedure by toning your intestinal tract's internal musculature for improved strength and resilience.

The following is a condensed set of instructions for performing an abdominal self-massage.

Abdominal Massage Technique	
Characteristic	Instructions and Considerations
Breathing	Breathe in deeply and slowly, in through the nostrils and out through the mouth. This will help develop your internal breathing power, sometimes known as your Chi (life force energy).
Location	Lying in bed or on a couch is ideal, but you may also massage while taking a warm, relaxing bath. Try to lay as flat as possible.
Hand Placement	Begin with your hands just above the groin area upon your lower abdomen. You can elevate your upper arms with small pillows to extend your reach and allow the hands a beneficial vantage point for pushing down. Work upwards to include the entire abdomen.
Pressure	Always apply light pressure and avoid compressing painful areas. Use your entire hand and coordinate your technique with natural breathing so you are not pushing down as your abdomen is expanding. It takes practice to develop your own sense of "touch" for massage but you should try to maintain consistency in the pressure used. Focus on feeling the softness of your intestines and organs beneath the skin, on natural contractions and movement, on blockages that diminish or go away, and on improved

Abdominal Massage Technique

Pressure (contd.)	"flow" within your entire digestive system.
Rhythm	Let your hands lift lightly when breathing in and push downward with mild to medium pressure when breathing out.
Technique	Use small circular motions, alternating clockwise and counter-clockwise, with your individual hands and then both together first towards each other and then away. Experiment with different patterns such as elongated ovals, zigzags, and small "rubbing" strokes. You can also vary which parts of your hands apply the pressure. Determine which movements benefit you most.
Time	Self-massage sessions should last between 15 and 30 minutes, with 5 minute "warm-up" phases to develop your rhythm and pressure and 5 minute "cool-down" phases to gradually ease the pressure applied.
Visualization	Water imagery is especially beneficial as it is constantly flowing, never occupying the same space twice, changing with each new wave to create a beautiful and unique expression of nature. The human body, mind, and spirit all resonate with the liquid formlessness of water. Imagine rising and drifting weightlessly on a vast, calm ocean.

Your intestines may not seem to respond to your massage treatments right away, as they may have become "sluggish" from years of eating bad foods and through loss of muscle tone. After practicing your technique for some time, you may begin to notice increased warmth from improved blood flow and a gradually lessening of tension in the abdominal area. As you attain this level of comfort and effectiveness, your massage treatments may eventually require less time for the same "return on investment" i.e. health benefits.

Abdominal massage also promotes inner harmony by relaxing the body. In our hyper-paced and work-focused society, many people walk around in a perpetual state of tension. This habit of constant nervous anxiety isn't good for us mentally, emotionally, nor physically—it can lead to the colon becoming chronically irritated by otherwise harmless stimuli whenever stress levels become elevated.

When done as a complement to a colon cleansing regimen, abdominal massage allows your body to become "centered" or balanced. You'll feel better physically and emotionally after a soothing massage session. Just think about how relaxed and stress-free you feel after receiving a deep-tissue back massage. The same benefits can be achieved from massaging your abdomen as well! In all of your health related exercises, keep in mind that a clean and healthy colon is one of the strongest assets you can have for preventing illness and disease.

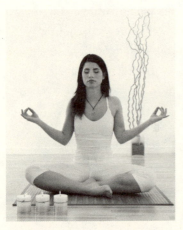

2. Daily Breathing

Practicing simple breathing exercises (such as slow, diaphragmatic breathing) and conscious muscle relaxation can help you clear your mind and calm your physical responses to stress. By relieving daily stress, you also relax the bowel. Deep, focused breathing also increases the oxygen content of the blood. Organs such as the colon depend on sufficient amounts of oxygen. Breathe in deeply through your nose for 4 seconds. Hold your breath for 16 seconds, and then release the air through your mouth gradually over 8 seconds. Repeat this exercise nine times to complete a session. Try to fulfill at least two sessions daily during the 6-Day Cleanse or whenever you feel stressed. It is also helpful to complete at least one session of deep breathing while sitting on the toilet before having a bowel movement.

3. Focus On Positive Emotions

It's easy to become wrapped up in today's busy world and focus on the negative instead of the positive (what's "wrong" with a colleague or a family member, rather than what's "right" with them). Negative stressors surround us, but we can't let ourselves be overwhelmed by them. If you're stressed, anxious, angry, or depressed, there's a very good chance your colon is "aware" of it. Stressful situations and emotions release hormones in the body that can have detrimental effects on our digestive health.

Surround yourself with positive energy. This could take many forms—listen to your favorite music, get a massage, and don't forget to smile. Smiling is contagious, and can positively affect everyone around you. Whether it's a close friend or a healthcare professional, find someone to talk to if you're having a hard time dealing with negative emotions.

Stress relief is critical! A tense state of mind will not help detoxify the colon and will actually contribute to colon toxicity. Do whatever it takes to decrease the negative energy forces in your life and replace them with stress-reducing, positive energy forces. **Live in the NOW!**

4. Get Plenty Of Sleep

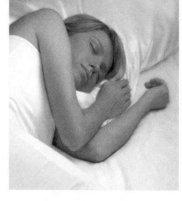

Getting enough sleep is difficult for many people. For Americans, this seems typical. We tend to "over-do it" in stressful environments such as work, and "under-do it" in life-sustaining activities such as exercise, healthy eating, and especially sleep. Working too hard and not getting enough sleep is the opposite of the ideal. Sleeping well is not a recommendation or suggestion—it's a requirement! The human body absolutely has to have time to rest and recuperate from its daily

> **DEFINITION**
>
> ***Pineal Gland:***
> Located between the brain's hemispheres in most vertebrates, this tiny endocrine gland secretes the hormone melatonin (derived from the amino acid tryptophan) and regulates sexual development, metabolism, and the circadian rhythm. Also known as the epiphysis cerebri or the "seat of the soul".

activities. Every animal knows this and instinctively rests after exertion or during the heat of the midday.

I believe it's important to retire to bed early (8:00 pm to 9:00 pm or 10:00 pm at the latest) to receive the beneficial regenerative magnetic fields of the earth.[43] I always advised my patients to go to bed 2 to 5 hours before midnight because this enables their bodies to increase the natural healing powers of the immune system necessary to restore health.

Sleeping well also aids the morning elimination cycle. Try to sleep in the darkest environment possible. When light hits the eyes, it disrupts the sleep rhythm of the **pineal gland** and production of melatonin and serotonin. This is why it's a bad idea to keep a nightlight burning in direct line-of-sight of the eyes. Besides ruining night vision, any amount of light while sleeping can keep you from getting sufficient rest!

5. Receive Regular Chiropractic Adjustments

The human body is an intricate design made up of millions of nerves executing our every move. One group of vital nerves is located in the Lumbar Spine region. These nerves are responsible for the control of bowel, urinary, and sexual functions in the body. When these nerves become overactive or underactive (from a herniated or bulging disc, a pinched nerve, or even a slight misalignment), all three of these important functions can suffer.

The Lumbar nerves control intestinal peristalsis, the wave-like contractions which help move waste through the body. Sometimes, pressure on these nerves can limit peristalsis and thus allow an onset of bowel dysfunction. When these nerves are affected, you may feel pain that spreads across your abdomen, nausea, or you may even lose control of your bowels.

Sometimes a simple spinal re-alignment is all that's needed to relieve the pressure on the nerves. Incorporating a routine chiropractic exam and spinal alignment into your health regimen can help keep this important group of nerves from being compromised. Your chiropractor can also detail some exercises to add to your routine which will strengthen and support the Lumbar Spine to help prevent these types of problems.

6. Acupuncture

Acupuncture is an alternative healing technique involving the insertion of specialized needles just beneath the skin along the body's meridian points. Acupuncturists seek to relieve pain and internal disharmony by stimulating these points to activate or balance the body's *Chi* or life force energy.

How Does Acupuncture Work?
First, the practitioner notes the patient's physical characteristics (quality of the eyes, tongue, and face) and overt symptoms (fever, chills, poor sleep patterns, perspiration, aches, and especially tenderness at specific points). Second, the practitioner inserts tiny needles approximately 3 to 5 millimeters beneath the skin and may apply heat (through moxibustion—the burning of an herbal substance at the exposed end of the needle), special herbs, micro-currents of electricity, mild pressure, or may simply leave the needles inserted. The needles typically remain inserted until the patient fully relaxes or until the meridian becomes balanced again.

The amount of time required for the procedure varies due to multiple factors—the patient's toxin buildup, level of relaxation or stress, and/or which meridian is affected and to what degree. However, the needles are far smaller in diameter than those used for a typical injection so pain is not really an issue. In fact, many patients describe a mild but pleasant tingling sensation during the procedure.

Acupuncture is intended to normalize the flow of energy back and forth between the points along the affected meridian. The meridian systems are typically named for the body's primary organs. Each point connects to an internal organ and is further classified as a Yin (female) or Yang (male) meridian. Most practitioners utilize a sort of standardized meridian system known as the Twelve Primary Pathways comprised of the bladder, gallbladder, heart, kidney, large intestine, liver, lungs, pericardium, San jiao (or abdominal cavity), small intestine, spleen, and the stomach.

How Can Acupuncture Help Me Detoxify Internally?

Acupuncture has been practiced for nearly 5,000 years and is receiving attention even in Western hospitals and clinics. Of particular interest is acupuncture's efficacy in alleviating symptoms of digestive difficulties such as bloating, nausea, Irritable Bowel Syndrome, diarrhea, and constipation.

When applied properly, acupuncture can even promote cleansing of the intestinal tract by helping it push out toxins. These harmful substances are trapped within the body until you remove them with special detoxifying supplements. Acupuncture can also be used to assist and open the body's elimination pathways. Moxibustion appears to be especially beneficial in this regard, as the mild heat expands the skin's pores to facilitate toxin release via natural perspiration. Alternately, the introduction of a mild electrical current through the meridians can likewise work to remove "obstructions" from neural messaging routes.

Once the body's organs begin communicating more effectively with the brain, the central nervous system, and each other, the absorption of vital nutrients and the elimination of waste can occur with greater ease. Detoxification experts are continually discovering how effective acupuncture is for complementing intestinal and body cleansing with their patients. Acupuncture predates modern science, so it's definitely worth trying as an additional means for maximizing your intestinal cleansing efforts!

Questions and Answers on the 6-Day Oxygen Colon Cleanse

Q. *Can I perform this cleanse and still carry on my daily activities?*

A. Yes, you can keep your regular routine while doing the cleanse. Just mix your gallon of ingredients and take it with you if you'll be away from home. For food, also take fresh fruit with you (you can clean and cut it up at home and put it into a sealed container). **Tip:** It's best to start a 6-Day Cleanse on a Friday or Saturday morning; this timing will give you access to a bathroom for longer periods, might relax you a bit, and will also let your body become accustomed to cleanse-related changes over the weekend. Continuing the 6-Day Cleanse should be manageable as long as you have a bathroom nearby.

Q. *Am I going to be stuck in the bathroom all day long?*

A. For the first few days, depending on your weight, you may need to stay close to a bathroom. Yet some people who have a large amount of compacted fecal matter may not have a bowel movement until the second or third day, though this delay is quite normal. Each person's results will be different. After all, you probably spent years (if not decades) slowly building up the toxic waste in your digestive system, so naturally it may take a little time to break it down. The average number of daily bowel movements during the cleanse is 3 to 7.

Q. *Will I lose weight during the 6 days of cleansing?*

A. This cleanse is not specifically intended for weight loss. While some people have reported weight loss ranging from 5 to 20 pounds when cleansing, this is not actual fat loss, but rather is due to the elimination of stored, hard-compacted fecal matter throughout the entire length of the intestinal tract.

Q. *How will I know when my bowels are clean and the compacted fecal matter is gone?*

A. Everyone's results on the cleanse will differ, depending on their diet, exercise patterns, and age, as well as physical and emotional stress levels. However, to ensure that you continue to stay as clean inside as possible, you should eat only live, raw fruits and vegetables and should completely eliminate as many environmental toxins as possible (see Part 2). Because the Standard American Diet (appropriately called "SAD") is so poor, you will need to cleanse on a continuous basis to help keep your entire intestinal lining clean. Therefore, I recommend a continued maintenance dose using a oxygen based cleanser 2 to 3 times weekly (especially after the consumption of red meat meals). Use your bowel activity as a guide. You will know how "clean" you are by the color, consistency, and frequency of your bowel movements. As your intestinal tract becomes progressively cleaner, the color of each succeeding bowel movement should be much lighter, and transit time (time from eating to elimination) should be shorter (12 to 16 hours). You should also be experiencing more frequent, softer, and smoother bowel movements. See Chapter 4 for details on normal stool evaluation.

Q. *How often should I repeat the 6-Day Oxygen Cleanse?*

A. Feel free to repeat the Oxygen Cleanse as needed. Factors will include what your typical diet consists of, the amount of toxins you expose yourself to daily, stressors in your life, and how well you feel generally. I recommend that you repeat the 6-Day Cleanse every 3 to 6 months if any of the following four conditions apply:

- Your diet regularly includes processed or fast foods, coffee, soft drinks, or alcohol.

- You're experiencing constipation or you feel compacted.

- You do not exercise regularly (that is, 3 times per week or more).

- You experience regular yeast infections, bloating, or gas.

Even if you follow my suggestions and eliminate toxins (as best you can) in your environment, improve your diet, and ramp up your exercise routine, you should still repeat the 6-Day Cleanse every 6 months, to help maintain optimal intestinal health.

Q. *What makes the Oxygen Colon Cleanse so different from other colon cleansing programs?*

A. The Oxygen Colon Cleanse is distinctly better than others primarily in its ability to clean the entire 25 to 30-foot length of the digestive tract. It's designed to clean it thoroughly, and reduce the amount of hard impacted fecal matter in the small and large intestines. This cleanse uses oxygen (O_2) from the fruit and singlet oxygen (O_1) in the cleanser to release useful oxygen into the bloodstream and bowel, and does so in a natural, nontoxic way. Estimates predict the average person has between 10 to 20 pounds of hard, compacted fecal matter lodged in their intestinal tract by the age of 40. Since the human intestinal tract is 25 to 30 feet long, if you were to cut it open and spread it out, the surface area would be the size of a tennis court. By using this cleanse, you can melt away or oxidize the compaction from the small intestine and the colon—safely and effectively. This is critical, because, as you know well by now, a clean intestinal tract is an essential step towards achieving optimal health.

Q. *What symptoms might I experience during the 6-Day Cleanse?*

A. During a cleanse, you may experience watery or gaseous stools, noisy bowel sounds, or some temporary cramping caused by gas.

Tip: To check the time it takes for food to go through your system (transit time), consume an entire ear of corn one evening with dinner, but do not consume any corn 3 days prior to testing. Record the time of the dinner meal. Then, watch for the corn to appear in your stool. As soon as you see the kernels in the stool, chart the day and time. This will be your current transit time. For accuracy I recommend repeating the corn test 2 or 3 times.

The Overnight "Quick Colon Cleanse"

Let's say you go out for dinner and over-eat and possibly over-drink. Eating too much at the dinner meal can wreak havoc on your colon, and make you feel miserable the next day. The steak, potatoes, wine, dessert, and everything else you consumed can sit in your intestinal tract for two to three days, because the improper mixing of foods causes the steak to putrefy, the carbohydrates to ferment, and the fats to turn rancid before they can be processed and then eliminated. Such an overload of food also depletes the enzymes needed to properly break the food down. In addition, most people are so eager to binge at a party meal they do not chew their food properly, thereby causing bigger chunks of food to move into the GI tract. I do not advise eating or drinking like this on a regular basis; yet, with our culture being the way it is, plus the poor quality of restaurant food, you may find it difficult to avoid an occasional dinner party where you eat too much or a night of indulgence at home. But if you do decide to splurge once in a while, it is better to get that garbage out of your system as soon as possible. An overnight "quick cleanse" is the easiest and fastest way.

Technique: Before bed, squeeze the juice of $^1/_2$ lemon (preferably organic) and add 1 teaspoon of organic apple cider vinegar into 16 ounces of purified or distilled water, and drink it along with 8 capsules of Oxy-Powder or other high-quality, oxygen-based cleanser. The next day, everything should be eliminated safely and effectively.

DOCTOR'S NOTE:
Because your stomach is full and therefore probably distended, you might experience temporary cramping after you consume your drink. If that happens, get up and walk around for 15 minutes or so to increase blood flow and let gravity pull the food down.

Tip: *Alcohol drinkers who use the overnight "Quick Colon Cleanse" report reduced hangover symptoms the next day and often have a renewed sense of energy.*

Can I Use Any Other Colon Cleansing Methods?

In general, colon cleansing options include oxygen-based cleansers, laxatives, herbal or fiber supplements, enemas, Bentonite or other cleansing clays, and colonic hydrotherapy. Colonic hydrotherapy and enemas are both mechanical methods of cleansing involving specialized equipment while laxatives and natural supplements (including oxygen-based cleansers) are usually administered orally or rectally.

It's important to be as informed as possible before you choose any particular method to cleanse your colon. I will do my best to objectively cover all the essentials of the major colon cleansing options including their advantages and drawbacks.

Since we already covered oxygen-based colon cleansers, let's review some of the other popular cleansing methods.

As you may know, colon cleansing methods are designed to remove the toxic waste polluting your intestines. Constipation is often one of the first signs of toxic buildup; and regular intestinal cleansing can help relieve your constipation symptoms and get things moving again in the bathroom.

However, a constipation remedy may not involve just colon cleansing, especially if the problem is addressed according to traditional medical guidelines. A good intestinal cleanser will attack the source of the constipation. Traditional constipation treatments (such as laxatives) may only temporarily relieve the symptoms and do nothing to address the compaction or heal the delicate intestinal tissue.

Can Laxatives Cleanse My Colon?

Laxative sales exceed $700 million annually.[44] Laxatives are usually the first thing that comes to mind when most people think about constipation relief, but they often bring serious health risks and they are not a valid or complete cleansing solution.

Many different types of laxatives are available and they utilize very different ingredients to achieve essentially the same result—eliminating blockage. Generally speaking, laxatives can be lumped into three categories: osmotic laxatives, stimulant laxatives, and bulk forming laxatives.

Osmotic Laxatives cause excess fluids to be drawn into the intestines in a slow process that can take up to a few days to increase the stool's fluid bulk. Basically, osmotics turn the stool into diarrhea so it's easier to pass. This type of laxative can also cause severe dehydration and electrolyte depletion from water loss, as well as cramping and bloating due to gas buildup during the initial waiting period.

EXAMPLES OF OSMOTIC LAXATIVES

Lactulose: Duphalac®[45], Kristalose®[46], and Actilax® (Lactulose)[47]

Sorbitol: Sorbilax®[48]

Polyethylene glycol compounds: MiraLAX®[49]

Magnesium Hydroxide (milk of magnesia): Phillip's® Milk of Magnesia[50], Dulcolax® Milk of Magnesia[51], and Freelax®[52]

Stimulant laxatives are made with harsh, often toxic chemicals or herbs that cause the intestinal muscles to spasm and contract. The popularity of stimulant laxatives stems from the fact they start working in a matter of hours. Unfortunately, stimulant laxatives can also cause the same diarrhea, dehydration, and gas-related pain as osmotic laxatives. If overused, stimulant laxatives can become incredibly addictive and cause long-term damage to the sensitive intestinal lining.

The intestines can quickly grow dependent on stimulant laxatives to trigger a "false" bowel movement, thus preventing normal intestinal contractions. This condition, known as "lazy bowel syndrome," ultimately results in a long-term battle with chronic constipation and the loss of bowel muscle tone and strength.

EXAMPLES OF STIMULANT LAXATIVES

Senna: Fleet® Liquid Glycerin Suppositories[53], Rite Aid® Senna Laxative[54], Traditional Medicinals® Smooth Move Herbal Stimulant Laxative Tea[55], ex-lax®[56], Senokot®[57]

Cascara Sagrada: Nature's Way® Cascara Sagrada Aged Bark[58]

Castor Oil: Swan® Castor Oil[59], Now® Foods Castor Oil[60]

Bisacodyl: Correctol® Bisacodyl Stimulant Laxative[61], Fleet Bisacodyl®[62], Dulcolax®[63], Gentlax®-S[64,] Rite Aid® Corrective Laxative Tablet[65]

Bulk-forming laxatives use highly absorbent materials (usually dead fiber instead of live fiber such as live fruits and vegetables) to increase overall stool mass. As the stool increases in size, the bowels are forced to expend more energy to force out the mass.

Fiber and increased stool mass are both usually good things, but bulk-forming laxatives can be dangerous since they have the potential to clog the bowels. Psyllium, used in most OTC (over-the-counter) fiber laxatives, is especially troublesome. Psyllium is one of the most common herbal ingredients in colon cleansers and especially in OTC fiber laxatives.

EXAMPLES OF BULK-FORMING LAXATIVES

Psyllium: Metamucil® Psyllium Fiber[66]

Guar Gum: Benefiber®[67]

Methyl Cellulose: Citrucel®[68]

> **DEFINITION**
>
> **Anaphylaxis:**
> An acute, multi-system allergic reaction that can lead to death in severe cases. Constriction of the airways (resulting in choking) is a common symptom.
>
> **Mucilage:**
> a thick, gooey type of substance produced by many plants.

There have been numerous reports of serious allergic reactions following the ingestion of psyllium products. These reactions include labored breathing, skin irritations or hives, and potentially life-threatening **anaphylaxis**.[69] Long-term use of products containing psyllium may also negatively affect absorption of certain essential vitamins and minerals such as iron. Perhaps most ironically, obstruction of the gastrointestinal tract has also been regularly cited in studies of patients taking psyllium products. These studies suggest this problem is especially common in constipation-prone individuals.

This brings us to herbal supplements claiming to cleanse the colon. Many of these products are actually just cleverly marketed bulk-forming laxatives!

Which Herbal Colon-Cleansing Ingredients Should Concern Me?

Over the last few years, the nation has been flooded with numerous infomercials on natural health, herbal colon cleansers, and detoxifiers. These may be natural, but virtually none of them are effective at ridding the colon of toxins. According to the National Library of Medicine, the National Institutes of Health, and similar organizations, many herbal colon cleansers are not only ineffective but can also put your health at serious risk.

The majority of these companies choose to include cheap and potentially dangerous ingredients in their formulations. Popular herbal ingredients to be especially wary of include Psyllium, Cascara sagrada, and Senna.

Many other potentially dangerous herbal combinations make their way into herbal cleansers, so be sure to research each and every individual ingredient in any herbal cleanser before putting it into your body.

Psyllium is a bulk-forming laxative that's high in both fiber and **muci-**

lage. The laxative properties of Psyllium (which is the seed of the fleawort plant, an Old World plantain) are due to the swelling of the husk when it comes in contact with water. When ingested, the resulting bulk stimulates a reflex contraction of the walls of the bowel. The Psyllium acts as a hard sponge as it works it way down. This often causes an emptying of the bowel.

While Psyllium may be marketed for short-term bowel emptying, it is not effective in fully cleansing the bowel, removing much of the toxic waste, or improving the long-term health of the intestinal walls.

Despite the claims of many manufacturers, use of laxatives or constipation relievers containing Psyllium (or its components or extracts), or ingestion of this "natural" herbal supplement, can be a potentially fatal decision. A recent search on *www.shopping.com* using the keyword "psyllium" revealed over 800 products and variants containing this ingredient.

Although most Psyllium-containing products offer direct-to-consumer sales, many can be found on the shelves of your neighborhood grocery store or pharmaceutical outlet. Psyllium has even been included in breakfast cereals marketed at reducing cholesterol by being "heart healthy." After all (or so the consumer is meant to think), if it's included in breakfast cereal, there can't be anything unsafe about it—right?

These products' manufacturers must be aware of the risk of using psyllium, as they include warnings on the labels similar to the ones below (chosen randomly from actual products).

"Psyllium Warnings

- Taking this product without adequate fluid may cause it to swell and block your throat or esophagus and may cause choking.
- Do not take this product if you have difficulty in swallowing.
- If you experience chest pain, vomiting or difficulty in swallowing or breathing after taking this product seek immediate medical attention.
- Keep out of reach of children.

- In case of overdose, get medical help or contact a Poison Control Center right away.

Allergy Alert: *This product may cause an allergic reaction in people sensitive to inhaled or ingested Psyllium.*

Ask a doctor before use if you have:
- A sudden change in bowel habits persisting for 2 weeks
- Abdominal pain, nausea or vomiting

Stop use and ask a doctor if: Constipation lasts more than 7 days or rectal bleeding occurs. These may be signs of a serious condition."

✚ DOCTOR'S NOTE:

A popular tactic used by companies selling herbal cleansers is to display pictures of "mucoid plaque ropes" deposited in the toilet. Don't let these disgusting strands of half-digested fiber fool you. No proof exists that these "mucoid ropes" are the built up toxic matter being excreted. I successfully duplicated this same mucoid substance in a lab by mixing Psyllium with white flour, hydrogenated oil, and plain water. You end up with a foul-looking but easily molded paste that will obviously take on the shape of anything including your colon.

Senna is an herbal stimulant laxative that is toxic to animal muscle tissue, yet this substance is a common ingredient in many herbal teas, weight-loss supplements, vitamins, and especially laxatives.[70] In fact, Senna is often prescribed as a "natural medicine" for curing constipation. Despite the alarming fact of its toxicity, senna continues to be included in hundreds of products while simultaneously causing a host of very serious health conditions, diseases, and even death in high enough concentrations.

When Senna becomes highly concentrated in the organs or bloodstream, through over-consumption by whatever means, this herb can lead to the recipient developing a variety of health problems. Senna seems to primarily affect body systems related to the blood and/or natural cellular functions but can also severely damage the liver.[71] Common diseases and conditions caused by Senna overuse or toxicity include:

- Decreased enzyme production
- Blood diseases
- Liver failure
- Musculoskeletal tissue damage
- Nervous system impairment
- Decreased energy production
- Unhealthy weight loss
- Severe diarrhea
- Diaper rash and blisters (in kids)
- Death of colorectal tissue (possibly leading to colon cancer)

Cascara sagrada is an herbal stimulant laxative which has been demonstrated through scientific processes to actually cause serious digestive problems, including worsening symptoms such as diarrhea and constipation rather than relieving them.[72] Other health conditions you can develop by using Cascara sagrada include:

- Acute Hepatitis (swelling of the liver)
- Liver damage
- Abdominal pain
- Rectal bleeding
- Lesions in the colon

Cascara is one of a group of herbal plants containing compounds called Anthraquinones—known cancer-causing agents. In other words, when lab animals receive this herb in sufficient quantities, tumors or colon cancer is often the result.[73] Remember—there is only a fractional amount of DNA differentiating human beings from many other mammals such as rats, primates, or even a household fly . . . so what can kill one animal can probably kill most.

You obviously don't want to ingest this herb or any of its derivatives. Take the time to seek out a product supporting your body's ability to cleanse and heal itself, rather than relying on a dangerous laxative that causes more harm than good.

Laxative products can be fairly inexpensive ($20 or so for a month's supply) to outrageously priced ($100 or more for a month's supply). Psyllium products usually require multiple steps—mixing different ingredients along with following a set regimen and can be time consuming and messy. I personally would rather take a couple of pills before I go to bed at night.

Many people state they have received benefit from bulk-forming laxatives so if you feel better using them, that's fine. I am not here to say what works for one person won't work for another, so it's up to you to make an educated decision. I'm just advising caution as you find out what works best for you. If you do however decide to use herbal laxatives, make sure the herbs are organically certified.

Are Enemas Effective for Cleansing the Colon?

Enemas are one of the oldest known techniques for cleansing the colon and treating constipation. People all over the world have used this technique for centuries.

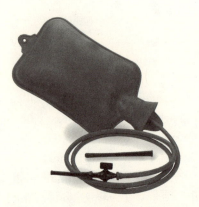

Fig. XIII: Enema Bag Kit

In its simplest form, an enema is a device inserted into the anus to inject fluid (usually water) from a holding bag into the rectum. This can be an effective method for removing waste that has become trapped in the lowest part of the colon, but it does very little to cleanse the entire intestinal tract.

Besides plain water, a number of different additives have been used in enemas. Herbal blends, oils, coffee, and diluted clay are just a few of the more popular examples.

So-called "dry enemas" are sometimes used to achieve a similar effect by injecting small amounts of sterile lubricant (such as non-medicinal glycerin) directly into the rectum using a disposable, non-hypodermic syringe. Dry enemas work a lot like a suppository but much more quickly. Some people prefer dry enemas to their wet counterparts simply because they aren't as messy. Less fluid going into the bowels means less fluid coming out of the bowels.

Enemas can be useful for occasionally treating an acute case of constipation. Their effectiveness, however, is somewhat limited and depends largely on the type of solution used in them. Because enemas are only able to loosen waste sitting at the last part of the bowels, they don't provide a long-term solution for preventing constipation or for removing intestinal toxins.

Many people are also uneasy with the idea of inserting something into their anus. Another thing to keep in mind is the fact that enemas can be uncomfortable. If administered incorrectly, an enema can cause serious damage to delicate tissues.

 DOCTOR'S NOTE:
In my practice I have recommended enemas consisting of organic coffee, organic herbs, and organic clay and have witnessed great results. Talk to your natural healthcare provider to see whether you can benefit from these types of enemas.

Is Bentonite Clay Effective for Cleansing the Colon?

Bentonite is heralded for its internal cleansing properties. This all-natural clay has been used to help individuals afflicted with several different symptoms of constipation (such as bloating and gas) and Irritable Bowel Syndrome. As a result, Bentonite clay has become a popular ingredient of many detoxification programs.

When taken internally, Bentonite clay may provide multiple benefits including:

- Detoxification of the liver
- Cleansing toxins from the colon
- Promoting a healthful bacterial balance in the digestive system
- Removal of heavy metals and chemicals after radiation treatments

- Boosting the immune system
- Supporting efficient cellular respiration
- Improving nutrient assimilation by the digestive system

This unique clay has very powerful *adsorptive* and *absorptive* properties. While the words may sound similar, they involve completely different processes.

Adsorption—The molecules comprising Bentonite clay are negatively charged. The molecules of toxins, harmful bacteria, and other disease-causing agents are positively charged. As the Bentonite clay traverses the colon, the negative ions attract the toxic, positive ions and bond to them. Ions on the outer edges of both molecules swap sides, causing an exchange reaction which electrically "satisfies" the molecules. The two molecules are thus bound together and the clay molecule literally absorbs the toxic molecule.

Absorption—Quality Bentonite clay possesses only 17 minerals. Chemically speaking, the fewer minerals found in a clay, the higher its potential

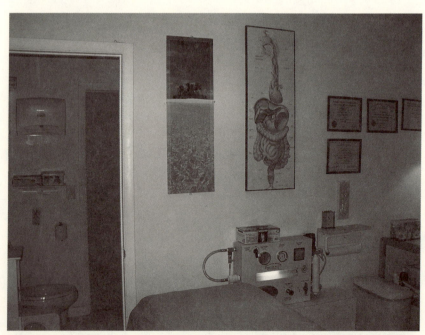

Fig. XIV: Colon Hydrotherapy Room

for absorption of other substances. The clay acts as a sponge as it absorbs the molecules that were initially exchanged and bonded in the adsorption process. The clay molecule takes the toxin molecule bonded to its exterior and assimilates it internally. Your body can then expel the toxin-filled clay molecules via normal bowel movements.

A word of caution however—Bentonite clay should not be taken if you are pregnant, of advanced age, or for at least two hours after taking other medications or nutritional supplements. No known side effects are associated with ingesting pure organic sources of this healing clay in the recommended amounts. However, Bentonite clay has not been subject to a longitudinal study focusing on its physiological effects in humans. It's always best to consult a qualified healthcare practitioner before taking any new supplement. Plus, you should take the time to conduct your own research and find a supplement with a history of safety as well as high standards of purity and effectiveness.

Is Colon Hydrotherapy Effective for Cleansing?

In many ways, colon hydrotherapy (or colonic irrigation), is like a supercharged enema. Although do-it-yourself kits are available for the adventurous, I recommend having this treatment administered by a properly trained, certified, and licensed professional at a private office, clinic, or spa. Most therapists are trained to massage the abdomen gently during the release cycle. This helps move the gas and waste trapped in the colon. It is wise to find a therapist using an FDA approved device with disposable speculums and tubing. The closed system is best. It is important for you to be checked for any possible risks before having this kind of treatment, especially in the case of a pregnant woman.

> ### CAUTION!
> *Colon hydrotherapy may not be suitable for people suffering from severe hemorrhoids, malignant polyps, active Inflammatory Bowel Disease, or active Diverticulitis.*

During a colonic hydrotherapy session, a therapist helps the client gently insert a small plastic tube called a speculum a few inches into the rectum. The speculum is attached to a plastic hose connected to the hydrotherapy machine. Then, warm, purified water enters the body and will slowly and gently begin to cleanse the colon. Depending upon your symptoms and health condition, your therapist may choose to add herbs, ozone, or special enzymes to the water to increase the benefits of the therapy.

As the water flows through your colon, it causes the muscles to contract and expand, encouraging the body to expel any undigested food, water, bacteria, gas, and mucous that have built up in the colon. This compacted toxic matter leaves your body by traveling through a separate evacuation tube leading back to the machine. Warm water flows gently in and out of your colon a few times in a typical session, which lasts between thirty and fifty minutes, depending on how you feel. The treatment process is painless and you may experience some warmth as the toxins are flushed from your body.

Colonic hydrotherapy is extremely effective at toxin removal, especially when supplemented with an oxygen-based cleanser. Many colon hydrotherapists now use oxygen cleansers in conjunction with regular hydrotherapy sessions to maximize the results.

> **REMINDER:**
> Some colon cleansing methods can often strip beneficial bacteria from the intestinal tract as they remove toxic waste. It's important to take a Probiotic supplement during and after any cleansing process to ensure the colon maintains a healthy population of beneficial bacteria. Ask your practitioner which Probiotic is best for you. In my experience, *Bacillus laterosporus* or *Bacillus coagulans* seem to work the best.

At this point, you've probably gathered that I support colon hydrotherapy and oxygen-based cleansers the majority of the time. I also recommend organic Bentonite clays or enemas on occasion and I wouldn't think of letting a friend or family member use anything else.

Colonic irrigation, oxygen supplements, Bentonite or other organic clays from the earth, and enemas are SAFE and EFFECTIVE when used correctly.

Here are two of many real, documented colon cleansing success stories!

"As a child, I had only one bowel movement per week. Therefore, I have struggled with constipation since childhood. In the beginning I went to medical doctors, but to no avail. In my twenties I still couldn't even go to the bathroom taking 8 prescription pills per night. When I was 32, I was introduced by my chiropractor to healthy alternatives. I am eternally grateful for this. I am now 45 and have come a long way since then.

From first hand experience, I feel that combining Oxy-Powder® with colonics has excellent results. My goal and my healthcare professionals' goal is for me to only have to do a colonic 2 times a year. I am to the point of only needing 1 colonic per month, and I am close to being able to do 1 colonic every other month. I gauge this with being able to have more than 1 movement per day - of which is a miracle of God from where I started. In the past 2 months, I have had 2 or more movements per day! God bless you and thank you for caring!"

Juli B., Broken Arrow, OK

I was inspired to enter this field about 30 years ago when I was so sick with candida/yeast overgrowth that I couldn't see to drive a car. My headaches were chronic and no painkillers were helping. I was blessed to be led to a wonderful chiropractor that had a colon hydrotherapist in his office. I began with a series of 12 sessions over the course of 6 weeks.

After the first session, my vision cleared. Two weeks later my headaches disappeared, never to return. Needless to say, I was reborn in health! Within the next few years, I left my real estate career behind to begin practicing Colon Hydrotherapy in 1992. I now teach at the International School for Colon Hydrotherapy, Inc. here in Florida.

Our graduates hail from over 11 different countries and we are proud of each one of them. They share our vision to help end the suffering and assist people in finding ways toward better health. Dr. Group's Oxy-Powder® is an integral part of our success. We suggest it to all of our people and we see amazing results!

Cathy Shea, President
International School for Colon Hydrotherapy, Inc.

Many other colon cleansing herbs and methods are widely available for your consideration. I have explained the most common methods above. Nevertheless, the purpose of this book is to focus on the causes of colon toxins and how to eliminate them. Therefore, I recommend you spend a lot of time studying Part II of this book and work hard at slowly reducing your exposure to everyday toxins.

Can I Do Anything Else To Help Keep My Colon Healthy?

Yes! You may find this surprising, but how you position your body on the toilet can affect the condition and health of your bowels. Sitting on a regular toilet seat is completely unnatural because it constricts the anal canal, resulting in incomplete evacuations. Think about it—toddlers often instinctively squat while moving their bowels. This is by far

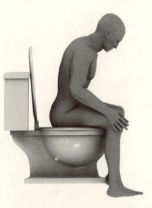

Unnatural Squatting

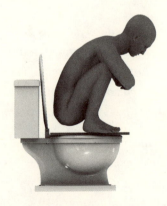

Natural Squatting

the healthiest position to adopt before having a bowel movement if you want to avoid constipation and maintain healthy intestinal function.

I recommend using a squatting platform to encourage relaxed and complete evacuation. These platforms may take a little getting used to, but you'll be happy once you discover your natural elimination position. To the right is a picture of a common platform. Many different platforms are available, so find one you will be comfortable with and that fits your toilet.

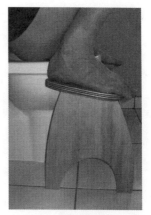

Fig. XV: Lillipad™

For more information, see "Squatting Platform" in the *Resources* section.

All of the cleansing methods I have shared with you up to this point require external materials. Did you know these methods are not the only way to purge harmful toxins from the body and stimulate normal bowel evacuation?

The human body actually has five natural elimination routes (only four in men). These are basically paths for purging harmful poisons out of the body:

1. Defecation (bowel movements)
2. Urination
3. Diaphoresis (sweating)
4. Respiration (breathing)
5. Menstruation (in women)

All five routes can effectively purge the body of toxins, provided that the body is at peak performance. Opening up these elimination routes can help reduce some of the burden from the colon. Therefore, it's important to have all the elimination routes in good working condition. This means you have to use them consistently and efficiently.

Exercise To Reduce Toxic Buildup

Exercise is the fastest and most effective way to open up elimination routes. Exercise can help reduce the toxic buildup in your colon, provide you with more energy, improve intestinal muscle tone, and promote efficient toxin neutralization, plus you'll feel increased vitality in almost no time! Exercise is a significant part of maintaining overall health and it can also drastically reduce your chances of developing serious diseases such as colorectal cancer.

Remember, exercise shouldn't over-exert your body. More importantly, it should be fun! You're more likely to stick with it if you engage in activities you really enjoy.

Here are a few great ways to exercise:

- Rebounding (my personal favorite)
- Long, leisurely bike rides
- Lively walking
- Hiking
- Swimming
- Martial arts
- Light jump-roping
- Rowing
- Pilates
- Yoga

If it's difficult for you to set aside time for a regular exercise routine, try to work it into your daily activities. Park in a space far away from the store entrance, take the stairs instead of the elevator, or ride your bike to work (if you can do so safely). The important thing is that you adopt an active lifestyle.

Mini–Trampoline Rebounding

Rebounding is an easy and fun exercise that is excellent for opening up all the elimination routes consistently and effectively. It's basically just jumping on a mini-trampoline in a very controlled but fun way. It's low-impact (so it won't damage joints), it's aerobic (it provides oxygen and we've seen how important oxygen is for the body), and has even been described by N.A.S.A. as the most efficient workout ever. If you think exercise is boring, tedious, or uncomfortable, you simply must try rebounding. Once you start bouncing, twenty or thirty minutes will have passed before you know it!

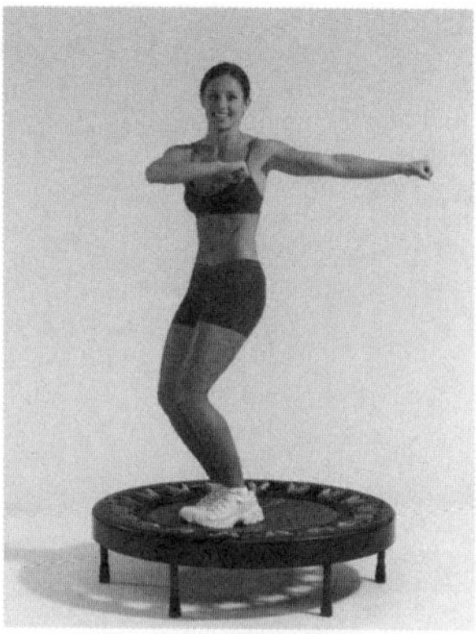

Health Benefits of Rebounding:

Fig. XVI: Mini-Trampoline by ReboundAIR™

- Opens up and supports all elimination routes
- Improves circulation of oxygen to organs (including the colon)
- Increases the functionality of the heart and lungs
- Strengthens the immune system
- Strengthens and drains the lymphatic system
- Boosts energy levels
- Lowers cholesterol
- Aids in digestion and massages the bowel
- Enhances metabolism
- May slow the aging process
- Reduces stress and anxiety

The following chart will help you identify ways to maximize the amount of toxins removed from your body.

Elimination Route	Ideas for Opening Up the Elimination Route
Respiration (Rapid Breathing from exercise) (Deep Breathing)	• Participate in aerobic activity for 30 minutes a day • Perform daily deep breathing exercises

Elimination Route	Ideas for Opening Up the Elimination Route
Diaphoresis (Sweating)	• Participate in aerobic or anaerobic activity for 30 minutes a day • Drink plenty of purified water • Treat yourself to a Far Infrared or Steam sauna session. (For more info, see "Heat Therapy" in the *Resources* section)
Defecation	• Have 2 to 4 bowel movements daily • Drink plenty of pure water • Eat only fresh organic fruits for breakfast each morning • Combine colon hydrotherapy with oxygen-based cleansers • Use a squatting stool with your toilet to encourage proper waste elimination • Don't delay when you have the urge to go
Urination	• Drink plenty of water • Don't delay urination when you have the urge to go. If you wake up during the night to urinate, it means this elimination route is partially blocked and you need to purge toxins. *See *Chapter 12—Dr. Group's Liver, Gallbladder, Parasite and Heavy Metal Cleanse*

Elimination Route	Ideas for Opening Up the Elimination Route
Menses	• Drink plenty of water • Avoid birth control pills because they automatically block the elimination of toxins through menses • Massage lower pelvic area during menses

Are you getting excited about cleansing your colon and opening up those elimination routes yet? You should be. The time has come for you to take charge of your health and your life! There's more to intestinal health than the occasional cleanse however. You have to be good to your colon every day! Are you ready to learn the best diet for your colon?

CHAPTER SIX

THE COLON DIET

"The doctor of the future will give no medicine, but will interest his patients in the care of the human frame, in diet and in the cause and prevention of disease."

-Thomas A. Edison

You're finally on your way to achieving optimal colon health! Hopefully, you plan to combine the benefits of colon hydrotherapy and oxygen colon cleansing to detoxify your colon. This is highly recommended. However, there's no quick fix! Simply purging toxins from your colon once in a while is not going to provide you

> **DEFINITION**
>
> **Biorhythms:** Biological cycles following an internal rhythm or pattern.

with the level of health and energy you need. Balanced dieting, getting regular sleep and sufficient exercise, reducing your daily toxin threshold, and maintaining a positive state of mind are required, as well. This may seem overwhelming at first, but I'm here to help you every step of the way. In the weeks and months to come, after your first cleanse, you'll be able to refer to the book's *Resources* section for a quick and easy guide, as well as notes you might jot down in any sections that seem particularly meaningful to you.

Let's learn about your body and its process so you can make healthy changes. Let's take a look at the **biorhythms** regulating our bodies.

The Human Body's Biorhythms

All creatures on this planet, including human beings, are naturally attuned to three daily body cycles. These cycles have precise and established hours set by the laws of nature.

BODY CYCLE #1:
THE ELIMINATION CYCLE

Begins around 4:00 AM and ends around 12:00 NOON.
During this cycle, the body naturally tries to purge itself of toxic waste materials and unnecessary salts, proteins, and acids. You should consume adequate amounts of fresh seasonal fruit (preferably organic or locally grown) during the elimination cycle. Not only does this supply the body with living matter to draw out unwanted substances, it also ensures the colon remains well hydrated and nourished. Fresh raw fruit provides the ideal ingredients for supporting the body's Elimination Cycle.

BODY CYCLE #2:
THE ENERGY CYCLE

Begins around 12:00 NOON and ends around 8:00 PM.
During the Energy Cycle, food and nutrients are processed and stored to

provide you with energy for your day. The best way to support your body during the Energy Cycle is to eat plenty of fresh raw vegetables (such as a salad) with a starch source to provide your body with the energy it needs to maintain its natural biochemical balance.

BODY CYCLE #3:
THE REGENERATION CYCLE

Begins from about 8:00 PM and ends 4:00 AM.
This is an opportunity for the body to take the time it needs to heal and regenerate. This is when the body should get quality sleep. During this cycle, the body assimilates all the foods that you consumed during the day and then processes the nutrients to regenerate itself cell by cell. If the sleep cycle is disrupted by irregular work patterns, night feeding of infants, travel across many time zones, or other factors, the body loses its ability to regenerate cells, which leads to their degeneration instead of regeneration.

What is the Best Diet Plan for the Health of My Colon?

I designed the following general diet suggestions based on the body's natural biorhythms. Understanding and following these principles are critical for first improving and then maintaining your health and vitality. Although this diet may seem tough at first, I would not be helping your colon or your body if I failed to tell you what they want and need to function properly.

For optimal health, all recommended foods should be certified organic or locally grown. This will help ensure their purity and nutritional content haven't been compromised by toxins such as pesticides, antibiotics, hormones, and other chemicals.

Raw organic fruits, vegetables, seeds, nuts, and sprouted grains provide the most nutrition to the body. Because they are not processed or treated (just gathered and cleaned), they provide the natural enzymes necessary for healthy digestion. If you were not raised on raw organic vegetables or foods, it may be difficult for you to make the transition from cooked, fried, and processed foods. Take it slowly and start by eating fresh fruit for breakfast every morning. After you've done that for a week or so, start eliminating one toxic food plus one toxic beverage every week until you have accomplished the goal of reducing your daily "toxic threshold." This process might last you 3 to 6 months, depending on how strict you are in following the plan. In Chapter 7, I explain precisely how to eliminate toxins from the foods you eat and the beverages you drink.

Drinking water or beverages with meals dilutes the digestive juices, which slows down the digestion process. Try to drink water between meals. If this doesn't suit your lifestyle, limit your water intake during a meal to less than 8 ounces. Drink only water with meals instead of milk, juice, soda etc.

You should eat 5 small meals daily to help regulate your metabolism. This might sound difficult, but when you think about it, it takes just a minute to peel and enjoy a banana or eat a handful of seeds or nuts.

Eat slowly and chew your food until it is a liquid-pulp before swallowing. This will allow your stomach to signal your brain, "hey I'm full now" so you avoid taking in excessive calories. You produce up to 32 ounces of saliva every day. Chewing your food will help your body absorb vital nutrients more thoroughly and rapidly due to the of enzymes secreted in your saliva. After food is liquefied in the mouth, the tongue will recognize the various flavors of each food and then send messages to the brain (which in turn orders production of the corresponding digestive juices needed to break down that food). Chewing your food well ultimately leads to more effective digestion and is also one of the best-kept secrets for losing weight.

Does any Combination of Organic Foods Create a "Perfect" Meal?

Consuming organic foods is a step in the right direction, but your body depends on the correct balance of food types. It's important to know how foods react with one another once they are inside the body. Many competing theories exist about the best food or diet combination to follow regularly. If any one person had all the answers, there would be a lot less disease in the world. So I will tell you what I have used, based on the biochemistry of the body, and on what has worked for me in my practice and my personal life. In the next few pages, I will cover the most damaging combinations of food, then I will present suggestions for five balanced meals I'm sure you will enjoy.

Mixing Proteins with Starches in a Meal Causes Colon Toxins

EXAMPLE OF STANDARD MEALS CONTAINING PROTEINS AND STARCHES:

Breakfast: Eggs, bacon, milk, sausage, or cheese combined with bread, potatoes, or tortillas.

Lunch/Dinner: Red meat, sandwich meat, or chicken combined with a baked potato, French fries, pasta, or bread.

When animal proteins and starches are metabolized, the end products are normally acidic. Your body should actually be slightly alkaline, not acidic. Your gastric juices contain three enzymes that act on proteins, fats, and milk; they are pepsin, lipase, and rennin, respectively. Protein digestion requires an acid environment initiated by the secretion of pepsin into the stomach. Pepsin splits the protein molecule to form hydrochloric acid. As the stomach becomes more acidic while digesting protein, starch digestion comes to an end. We may say those conditions which are optimum for protein digestion, exclude starch digestion. Worse, the introduction of the starch almost neutralizes the acid, thus deactivating the enzymes and creating the climate for putrefaction and fermentation. Non-starchy vegetables make for the best combinations with proteins. Refer to the food chart on the following page.

Combine proteins with non-starchy vegetables.

Starchy Vegetables and Grains	Non-Starchy Vegetables (Best Combination with Proteins)	
• Bagels	• Alfalfa sprouts	• Mushrooms
• Beans	• Artichokes	• Okra
• Bread	• Asparagus	• Onions
• Corn	• Bamboo shoots	• Peppers
• Lentils	• Broccoli	• Radishes
• Muffins	• Brussels sprouts	• Rutabaga
• Pasta	• Cabbage	• Sauerkraut
• Potatoes	• Carrots	• Snow peas
• Tortillas	• Cauliflower	• Spinach
• White rice	• Celery	• Summer Squash
• Winter squash (butternut, acorn)	• Eggplant	• Tomatoes (fruit)
	• Green beans	• Turnips
• Yams	• Leafy lettuce	• Water chestnuts
	• Leeks	• Zucchini

Mixing Acid Foods with Starches in a Meal Causes Colon Toxins

Example: Bread, pasta, rice, etc. + any acid fruit or fruit juice

The digestion of starches begins in the mouth with an enzyme called ptyalin (pronounced tie-uh-lun). Saliva, which is high in ptyalin, is secreted by the salivary glands and reduces starch to maltose, which in turn is reduced in the intestines to dextrose. Ptyalin will not activate in a mildly acidic or strong alkaline environment. The acid in regular vinegar, grapefruit, lemons, or other sour fruits will completely stop the action of ptyalin, resulting in a poorly digested meal. These meals will likely ferment, producing toxic byproducts as well as decreasing the nutritional value. Basically you shouldn't mix acids and starches during meals.

Mixing Acids with Proteins in a Meal Causes

Colon Toxins

Example: Meat + any acid fruit or fruit juice

Pepsin (an enzyme that digests protein) will act favorably in an acid environment. Therefore, you might think the addition of more acids, such as citrus fruits, might improve the digestive process. This is not so! The addition of citrus or other acids stops the secretion of the gastric juices necessary for protein digestion. Either the pepsin will not be secreted in the presence of an acid, or the acidic environment will destroy the pepsin. Any acid (say, vinegar or lemon) on a salad, when eaten with a protein meal, stops the production of hydrochloric acid since the pepsin interferes with protein digestion. An exception to this rule should be noted: acids can be combined with nuts and seeds because the high fat content of these foods will postpone gastric secretion until the acids have been assimilated into the body. Therefore, use raw nuts or seeds (not roasted or salted) with salads to neutralize the acids typically found in salad dressing.

Eating Meat with Cheese or Milk in a Meal Causes Colon Toxins

If two different types of high proteins are eaten together, the amount of digestive secretions for each might stop the action of the other. In other words, your body can modify the digestive process to accommodate each food. Suppose milk was eaten with meat—this would initiate a highly acidic reaction and upset the proportions of pepsin and lipase acting on the meat. Both proteins would not be fully digested, leading to the development of colon toxins.

What are some alkaline foods for neutralizing acid-forming foods?

Alkaline foods should be consumed 80 percent of the time. These foods aid in digestion, neutralize acids, and help restore the body's natural alkaline state. The following foods should always be eaten fresh, raw, or lightly steamed and should be locally or organically grown. Although some fruits are classified as acid fruits, once they are broken down in the body they convert body fluids to an alkaline state.

Highly Alkaline Fruits and Vegetables (Best Option)		Other Alkaline Fruits and Vegetables	
• Almonds • Avocados • Blackberries • Carrots • Celery • Chives • Cranberries • Currents • Dates • Endive • Figs • Grapes (sour)	• Kale • Plums • Pomegranates • Prunes • Raisins • Raspberries • Romaine • Soybean sprouts • Spinach	• Alfalfa • Apples • Apricots • Artichokes • Bamboo shoots • Beans (snap, string, wax, navy) • Beet leaves • Beets • Berries (most) • Bok Choy • Broccoli • Cabbage (red, white, Savoy, Chinese) • Cantaloupe • Celery • Cherries (sweet/sour) • Chicory • Coconuts • Cucumbers • Eggplant • Garlic	• Grapefruit • Honeydew • Horseradish • Kelp • Leeks • Lemon • Mangoes • Nectarines • Okra • Onions • Oranges • Organic Apple Cider Vinegar • Papayas • Parsnips • Pears • Pineapples • Pumpkins • Romaine lettuce • Tangerines • Tomatoes • Turnips • Watermelon

General Recommended Diet Plan

Now that you've learned the basics about food mixing and optimal combinations, read on to find a ready-made diet plan that you can start today. This is no bland, uninspiring diet, either. The foods I've included (if prepared properly) are so loaded with energy and flavor, you won't ever want to return to eating the high-fat, processed foods we've become so accustomed. Eating 5 balanced meals at the recommended times each day can help restore the health of your colon, and consequently restore and enhance your overall well-being.

DOCTOR'S NOTE:
I recommend getting a full evaluation by a qualified natural healthcare provider, as well as having a food allergy test performed. The Colon Diet is a general diet plan based on the body's biorhythms as well as my clinical experience. Every person should have a custom plan–one developed to meet their specific dietary needs

MEAL #1 OF THE DAY: BREAKFAST
Have breakfast between 4 a.m. and 9 a.m. Eat organic fresh fruit or drink freshly squeezed fruit juice. Eat or drink only fruit. Try to mix up the fruits during the week. For example, do not eat bananas every morning. Try melons now and then, as they are one of the easiest foods to digest. Melons actually proceed directly to the intestines after being consumed. If they are held up in the stomach by other foods, they will decompose quickly and ferment. A melon is a great way to start the day. You can eat a different variety of fruits throughout the whole morning, but never mix sweet fruits with acid fruits. It's okay to mix sweet with subacid or acid with subacid (see below). Eat as much as you want until you are full. Remember, we are supporting the body's Elimination Cycle.

> ACID FRUITS (These fruits have the greatest detoxification power): Lemons, oranges, pineapples, strawberries, grapefruit, kumquats, tomatoes, tangerines, lime, sour grapes, and sour apples

SUBACID FRUITS: Apricots, apples, pears, nectarines, sweet plums, cherries, mangos*, raspberries, kiwi, blackberries, blueberries, and cranberries

SWEET FRUITS: Bananas, papaya, dates, prunes, sweet grapes, cantaloupe, coconuts, mangos*, peaches, pears, watermelon, dates, figs, pomegranates, honeydew melon, and persimmons
*Mangos are both sweet and subacidic.

MEAL #2 of the day: MID-MORNING SNACK
(Should be eaten halfway between breakfast and lunch)
For a nice brunch, you can snack on 1 of the following items:
Choose A, B, C, or D. (For example, you might eat A on Mondays, B on Tuesdays, C on Wednesdays, and so on.) Remember to chew your food well before swallowing.

A—RAW NUTS OR SEEDS: My favorite! It's said that a handful of seeds will provide the body with 12 to 14 hours of energy. Many people have reported that after eating seeds for their mid-morning snack for three months, they noticed a 300 to 400 percent increase in their energy levels. Make sure your seeds or nuts are raw—roasted seeds have lost their life force. For more flavor, you can mix in some hempseed oil, garlic juice, balsamic vinegar, or organic apple cider vinegar.

CHOOSE FROM AMONG THE FOLLOWING DELICIOUS SEEDS OR NUTS: Almonds, cashews, pumpkin seeds, Brazil nuts, pistachios, sunflower seeds, flax seeds, hemp seeds, wheat berries, grape seeds, hazelnuts, pine nuts, squash seeds, sesame seeds, macadamia nuts, and walnuts. Siberian cedar nuts have one of the highest life-force energies and are the most nutritious and medicinally valuable pine nuts in the world; you can purchase these from *www.energyoflife.ca*. I also recommend that you read the book, *Anastasia* by Vladimir Megre, which will open your eyes and touch your soul.

B—ORGANIC SUPER GREEN FOOD SUPPLEMENT: Supplement with a high-quality green powder mix (wheat grass or a chlorella supplement), in a 20-ounce glass of purified water and add 1 teaspoon of organic Apple Cider Vinegar. This is fast and easy and provides your body with the nutritional value of five full salads!

C—ORGANIC GOJI BERRIES: If you're not familiar with the remarkable health benefits of Tibetan goji berries, do yourself a favor and try them. They pack more nutritional value into each bite than just about any other food.

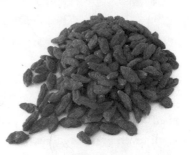

Fig. XVII: Organic Goji Berries

D—ORGANIC AVOCADO: Cut your avocado and sprinkle with fresh ground black or white pepper and squeeze fresh lime juice over it before eating. The pepper will help speed up your metabolism and the avocado contains the enzyme lipase. Foods containing lipase are the ones with naturally occurring "good fat." New research from UCLA indicates organic avocados are the highest fruit source of lutein (a carotenoid that helps prevent eye disease) among the 20 most frequently eaten fruits.[74] In addition, researchers found that avocados have nearly twice as much vitamin E as previously reported, making them the highest fruit source of this powerful antioxidant. Avocados also contain four times more beta-sitosterol than any other fruit. Some studies have found that the avocado's beta-sitosterol content, combined with its monounsaturated fat content, helps to lower cholesterol levels.

MEAL #3 of the day: LUNCH
Vegetables + Starchs
Have lunch between 11:30 a.m. and 1:30 p.m. Choose 2 to 3 alkaline vegetables (no acidic ones) and combine with a salad of fresh spinach, mixed lettuce, and greens (such as arugula, beet greens, or kale). Organic

> **DEFINITION**
>
> *Ezekiel Bread:* Refers to a Biblical edict (Ezekiel 4:9) to bake bread with ingredients such as wheat, barley, beans, lentils, millet, and fitches, and without artificial ingredients.

salad dressing or a mixture of oil and organic apple cider vinegar are excellent complements. Select only the red or dark-green leafy types of lettuce. Iceberg-type lettuces are usually hybrids and contain virtually zero nutritional value. Spinach (and baby spinach) is an excellent source of nutrients, and besides that it tastes great in salads. Mix some raw seeds or nuts of your choice into the salad.

CHOOSE TWO TO THREE STARCHY FOODS FROM BELOW TO ACCOMPANY YOUR SALAD: Potatoes (red, baked), cooked barley, beans, pumpkin, squash, **Ezekiel bread**, sprout bread, seven grain bread, whole grain pasta, lentils, millet, oatmeal, sweet potatoes, rice (brown or wild), rye, sauerkraut, chick peas, beets, or cauliflower. If it can be eaten raw it is best, otherwise steam, boil, or bake.

MEAL #4 of the day: MID-AFTERNOON SNACK
(Should be eaten halfway between lunch and dinner)
These options will be the same as your mid-morning snack. Choose A, B, C, or D (see the Meal #2 on page 120). (For example, you might eat A on Mondays, B on Tuesdays, C on Wednesdays, and so forth)

MEAL #5 of the day: DINNER
Vegetable + protein + fat
It's best to have dinner between 6 and 8 p.m. As with lunch, eat a large, fresh vegetable salad (with only alkaline vegetables) before anything else. Mix 2 tablespoons of organic flaxseed oil, cold-pressed olive oil, hempseed oil, or grape seed oil into your salad. This dressing will provide more flavor as well as the essential fatty acids your body needs.

Although you need to pick one protein source for dinner, I strongly recommend you avoid meat. If you absolutely must have meat on occasion, limit it to one serving per week and make sure it's organic. Meat should come from animals raised without harmful antibiotics and hormones.

SOME GREAT SOURCES OF HEALTHY PROTEIN
(make sure they're organic):
- Cold-water fish (cod, halibut, sole, haddock)
- Cottage cheese
- Other organic cheeses
- Eggs
- Fermented soy
- Hemp milk
- Lamb
- Legumes*
- Rabbit
- Range-fed beef or buffalo (bison)
- Raw goat or cow milk
- Veal
- Wild game (deer, squirrel, duck, quail, etc.)

*Legumes include beans and peas, and can be a good source of protein if eaten with mixed vegetables (in a salad) or with a complete protein (seeds, nuts, meat, and eggs). On their own, legumes are incomplete proteins and contain only certain amino acids.

If you want a little extra seasoning for your meal, Celtic or Himalayan sea salt is an excellent substitute for regular table salt and Braggs™[75] Liquid Aminos blend can perk up any dish!

Make sure you don't overdo eating at dinnertime. Let your appetite be your guide and (I'll say it again) chew your food thoroughly!

PART 2
HOW TO LIVE IN A GREEN, TOXIN FREE ENVIRONMENT

CHAPTER SEVEN

HOW TO REDUCE INTESTINAL TOXINS FROM FOOD AND BEVERAGES

In this chapter, I will go over the most common intestinal toxins found in the foods and beverages you eat and drink. These toxins include genetically modified foods, pesticides (used to treat the crops), meat and dairy, soy, white flour, table salt, MSG (Monosodium Glutamate), microwaved foods, refined sugar, artificial sweeteners, caffeinated drinks (colas, coffee, etc.), and alcohol. At the end of each category, I provide you with a quick reference chart for the easiest way to eliminate or reduce your daily exposure to these toxins. Remember, preventing toxins from entering your body is the

> **DEFINITION**
>
> **Synthesize:**
> To artificially create something by combining individual elements.
>
> **Synergistic:**
> Used in this case to describe the compounds in living organisms that work together so the total effect is greater than the sum of the individual parts.

real secret to health! Some of the content may seem overwhelming, sickening, or even shocking, but this is necessary for your full understanding of each subject area.

Because we are accustomed to our dietary habits, I recommend eliminating these toxin-producing substances at your own pace. Some people try to eliminate everything at once but it's easier to eliminate or greatly reduce 2 or 3 toxin producing compounds each week. For example, you might start by eliminating microwaved food and white flour during week 1 and soy and MSG in week 2.

Every journey begins with a first step, and you are obviously ready to embark on your transformation in health or you would not be reading this book. Set realistic goals and be patient and I will show you how to achieve optimal health.

Openly consider the foods you put into your body. How much of your diet consists of healthy, nutritious food that helps your mind and body grow and thrive? How much of your diet includes processed foods filled with toxic chemical additives and preservatives?

Even "healthy" foods such as fresh fruits and vegetables are not always as safe and nutritious as you might believe. Thanks to irresponsible commercial farming techniques that depend on chemical fertilizers, pesticides, and hormones to grow crops on already overworked land, a large percentage of today's produce supply has become saturated with toxins and has very little nutritional value.

Everything was fine until large corporations began creating their own "improved" foods, forcing them to mature unnaturally and boosting their size for increased profits. When you take something from nature and you manipulate or **synthesize** it, this substance loses its **synergistic** qualities, and becomes almost useless to the body. The once-living object becomes just another foreign chemical or altered structure our bodies interpret as "dead" or "toxic."

Foods grown in nature are overflowing with life-giving energy. The manufactured foods intended to replace them do not possess this essential quality. It is impossible for these false foods to nourish our bodies because they are nutritionally void. *The energy or life force in food is the key to maintaining a healthy body.* If you can remember the simple formula, "Live food equals life and dead food equals death" you have taken an important step towards achieving a healthy colon and body.

> **DEFINITION**
>
> *Enzymes:*
> Special proteins produced by living organisms that act as biochemical catalysts.
>
> *Detoxify:*
> To cleanse the body of accumulated toxins.

How real is the difference between raw, living foods and dead foods that have been processed and cooked? It's as real as the change between a cow munching grass in a field and bloody cow parts wrapped in cellophane with an expiration date in a grocery store.

What are Live Foods?

Raw fruits, vegetables, seeds, nuts, and whole grains are all good examples of live foods. The human body depends on these kinds of foods for energy to constantly restore and maintain health.

What are Dead Foods?

By contrast, dead foods have been robbed of their nourishing vitality. Also, these foods are laced with toxins from the artificial conditions employed to grow, process, and prepare them for sale. For instance, pasteurization uses heat to kill the valuable live **enzymes** in dairy products. Without these enzymes, dairy products can be toxic to your body, leading to allergies and other immune system problems.

If heat can kill the enzymes in raw foods during pasteurization, it will also kill them in the foods we cook. Raw living foods (loaded with nutrients and active enzymes) are much healthier than over-cooked foods devoid of any nutritional value. Fresh, raw foods such as fruits and vegetables help **detoxify** the colon and body naturally, thereby preventing disease.

> **DEFINITION**
>
> ***Refined:*** Meaning, a substance has undergone chemical or mechanical manipulation prior to consumption.

More than half a century ago in his book *Prescription for Energy,* Charles de Coti-Marsh explained, "By eating live foods you create a live body. Live foods contain essential nutrients the body needs to create and maintain energy. Dead foods advance age, decrease ability, and decrease energy ... they are useless when dead, exposed to air, soaked with water or unduly dried."

Convenience foods (pre-cooked, processed, or **refined**) not only lack these life-sustaining nutrients but they're loaded with chemicals that accumulate in the colon, thus forming toxic residue. If this toxic sludge sits in the colon long enough, it will work its way through the intestinal lining and back into the bloodstream contributing to the onset of life shortening diseases.

A good way to prevent disease would be to start eating plenty of raw foods... right? Well, yes and no. A diet consisting of nutrient-rich raw foods is a smart and healthy choice, but surprisingly, many of these foods are losing their life-sustaining qualities due to modern manufacturing techniques.

What Happened to All the Nutrients?

Discouraging trends in agriculture are leading to nutrients being stripped from the land and crops. The problem lies with the poor condition of our ecosystem, our appetite for cheap foods, plus the advent of genetically modified foods. Healthy soil contains insects and other life forms that crawl around, die, and thus replenish nutrients. Nowadays, however, crops are sprayed with pesticides that kill the insects and also poison our food and soil.

Land should be given time to "rest" and replenish itself after certain harvests. However, rotating crops is rarely practiced anymore. Large companies are buying up farmland and using chemical fertilizers to force-produce crop after crop to amplify yields for increased demand. The ultimate result of these profit-driven farming practices is toxin-laced crops with little nutritional value, not to mention the economic hardship of small-production farmers who cannot compete with multi-million dollar corporations.

> **DEFINITION**
>
> **Niacin (Nicotinic acid):**
> Part of the Vitamin-B complex made from the oxidation of nicotine.

For example, twenty years ago a half-pound of spinach contained 50 milligrams of iron. A half a pound of spinach today contains just five milligrams! A recent study commissioned by the *Globe and Mail* and CTV news in Canada revealed shocking facts about the current nutritional value of various crops. The study analyzed seven nutrients in 25 different fruits and vegetables. The findings were less than encouraging.[1]

Food (1951-1999)	Nutrient and Amount of Change (Percentage)[2] [Note: Negative Changes are Highlighted]						
	Calcium	Iron	Vitamin A	Vitamin C	Thiamine	Riboflavin	Niacin
Apple	20.0	-55.3	-41.1	16.0	-75.0	-66.7	-30.0
Banana	-23.8	-41.7	-81.2	-13.0	0.0	-100.0	-1.4
Broccoli	-62.8	-33.9	-55.9	-10.1	-40.0	-42.9	-2.7
Onion	-37.5	-52.9	-100.0	-54.8	56.9	-41.2	135.3
Potato	-27.5	-58.6	-100.0	-57.4	-14.6	-50.0	44.9
Tomato	-55.7	-18.8	-43.4	-1.6	0.0	21.8	46.3

The potato, for example, has increased its **niacin** levels over the past 48 years, but it has lost the following:

- 14.6% of its thiamine
- 28% of its calcium
- 50% of its riboflavin
- 57% of its Vitamin C
- 59% of its Iron
- 100% of its Vitamin A

> **DEFINITION**
>
> **Bioengineering:**
> An alteration produced by modifying the genetic structure of a biological process or organism.

Most troubling was the analysis of broccoli—its content for all 7 nutrients had decreased, and its calcium had diminished by a whopping 63 percent![3]

 DOCTOR'S NOTE:
Professor Tim Lang of the Centre for Food Policy in London states you would have to eat eight modern oranges to obtain the same amount of Vitamin A your grandparents enjoyed from just one! Poor nutrient content in soil is not our only worry though. As if the damage caused by pesticides isn't enough, crops are now being altered through genetic modification until they are no longer "natural" at all!

How Do Genetically Modified Foods Cause a Toxic Colon?

Genetically modified organisms (GMOs) come from plants or animals that have received new genetic material to achieve various results thought to be desirable. Experiments with the genetic makeup of diverse plant crops have led to resistance to pesticides, herbicides, and insecticides, enhanced levels of nutrients, and even tolerance to extreme weather conditions. Common products derived from genetically modified plants include cottonseed oil, soybeans, cocoa beans, canola, and corn. Genetically altered crops are taking over farmland at an alarming rate. **In 2006, United States GMO crops reached just shy of 135 million acres, with the total global area exceeding 250 million acres!** [4]

While enhanced nutrients and built-in pest resistance may seem to be a step in the right direction, in actuality the foreseeable future for GMOs is alarming. Scientists are **bioengineering** plants to manufacture pharmaceutical compounds (a technique known as "pharming"), trees which yield fruit and nuts much earlier in the season than they would naturally, plants that produce new kinds of plastics, and fish that reproduce more rapidly. Margaret Wertheim, in a 2002 article in *LA Weekly*, expressed fears that "Quietly and stealthily, our fields are being turned into industrial factories. *This is potentially the most dangerous technology since* *nuclear power,* yet we have no way of finding out what is being done."[5]

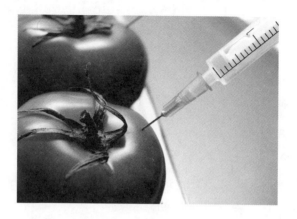

In 1994, the Flavr Savr® tomato (engineered to resist rotting) was the first genetically modified food reviewed and *approved* by the U.S. Food and Drug Administration for human consumption. FDA-employed scientists warned that altered products such as the Flavr Savr® could create toxins in food and trigger allergies. Shockingly, the FDA approved the "Frankenstein" tomato anyway with claims, "… the Flavr Savr passed muster so well that the rigor of its testing will not have to be repeated for other bioengineered foods."[6] The FDA also suppressed a report that described lesions being created in the stomachs of mice that had eaten the Flavr Savr®. As a matter of fact, "Seven out of forty rats tested died within two weeks for unstated reasons."[7]

How to Eliminate Toxins from GMO FOODS

- Buy organic foods! Organic foods are grown naturally, without using genetic modification.

- When eating soy, use organic fermented sources such as natto (fermented soybeans), tempeh, miso, tamari, or tofu. If soy is not labeled "organic", it is most likely genetically modified.

- Avoid canola oil and cottonseed oil. Make sure you read ingredient lists to ensure these oils were not used for food processing. Replace them with organic sources of virgin

How to Eliminate Toxins from GMO FOODS (contd.)

coconut oil, olive oil, or grapeseed oil, available from markets specializing in organic and whole foods.

- Corn and popcorn are usually genetically modified. Use organic varieties only.

- Zucchini and yellow squash are now being genetically modified for color and size. Use organic or locally grown sources.

- Avoid all products containing Aspartame as it is genetically modified and extremely toxic.

- Most meat and dairy products come from animals fed genetically modified feed. Buy organic, range fed, hormone and antibiotic-free meat and dairy products.

- Become politically active! Send letters to grocery chain executives and talk to the store managers at your local supermarkets. Ask them to stop buying GMO foods and to replace them with organic or 100% natural, toxin free foods.

- For an extensive list of foods and brands containing GMO's, visit www.truefoodnow.org

"So, wait just a second," you might be thinking, "aren't raw foods supposed to be beneficial to our health? If we can't count on raw fruits and vegetables to be pure sources of nutrition, how are we supposed to obtain the energy necessary for life?"

The answer lies in choosing organically grown or locally grown (farmer's market) foods. Even better, you should grow your own food organically in a backyard garden, provided you don't live near sources of pollution such as refineries, heavy industry, or freeways. What does organic mean? The United States Department of Agriculture (USDA) National Organic

Program defines organic food production as "… products produced under the authority of the Organic Foods Production Act. The principal guidelines for organic production are to use materials and practices that enhance the ecological balance of natural systems and that integrate the parts of the farming system into an ecological whole. Organic agriculture practices cannot ensure that products are completely free of residues; however, methods are used to minimize pollution from air, soil and water."[8]

> **DEFINITION**
>
> *Aspartame:*
> An artificial sweetener marketed under several brand names, Aspartame is commonly used in more than 5,000 consumer products such as diet colas, candy, chewing gum, and baking goods. The substance has been linked in several studies to higher incidence of tumors and lesions of the brain, cancer, and even DNA damage.

It's becoming increasingly common to see organic fruits and vegetables at many grocery stores but difficult to find quality organic meat, but it's well worth the search. You can purchase organic beverages, such as all-natural juices made from organic fruits and vegetables, now as well. Most likely, you can find a local farmer's market in or near your city, especially near rural areas. A farmer's market is the best place to buy your food because it is grown in your local environment and picked ripe, plus it supports local, small-production farmers.

You might be saying, "I know organic foods are good for me, but they're too expensive." My response is—how much do you think your health is worth? By comparison, how much do you spend each year on new clothes, personal grooming, or even on a $3.50 fresh latté every morning?

Now, let's examine other toxic food products you can avoid, their effect on your colon, and why you should begin slowly eliminating these harmful substances from your diet.

How Do Pesticides in Food Cause a Toxic Colon?

Pesticides, by definition, are used to rid an area of perceived "pests" such as insects, fungi, or weeds. Pesticides can take the form of chemicals, bacteria, or viruses. Used on crops to kill annoying invaders, pesticides often remain in the cultivated food products. When humans consume contaminated foods, these chemicals (which are strong enough to kill insects and other organisms) accumulate in the colon and slowly poison the body.

Important Facts about Pesticides

- "Most of the food produced for human consumption is grown using pesticides."[9]

- "Industrial contaminants (such as dioxins, PCBs, and mercury), microbial contaminants (such as E. coli), and natural contaminants (such as aflatoxin) [can also be found in foods]."[10]

- "In 1994, 62 percent of all food samples tested by the U.S. Department of Agriculture's Pesticide Data Program (PDP) had detectable levels of at least one pesticide."[11]

- "PDP data from 1994-96 … [stated 25] percent of the samples had detectable levels of carcinogenic pesticides, and 34 percent" possessed detectable levels of **neurotoxic** pesticides.[12]

- Kids who consume non-organic foods can retain as much as 8 times as many organophosphates[13] and this overload can cause birth defects, childhood leukemia and other cancers, brain tumors, neuromuscular damage, metabolic impairment, asthma and other bronchial disorders, digestive difficulties, and a variety of developmental delays.[14]

DEFINITION

Neurotoxic: Any toxic substance (manufactured or natural) that can adversely affect the neurological structure or function of the human nervous system (including the brain).

In an effort "…to protect the health of the consumer and ensure fair practices",[15] the Food and Agriculture Organization of the United Nations (FAO) and the World Health Organization (WHO) jointly formed the Codex Alimentarius Commission (CAC) in 1963. The intent of the 172 nations originally involved was to create a set of international food standards, guidelines, and codes of practice promoting food safety.

Despite their stated focus on "consumer protection," the Codex Commission approved seven of the most toxic chemical compounds known to man for use as pesticides in the production of foods! Collectively these chemicals are often referred to as Persistent Organic Pollutants (POP's) and are used in the production of a variety of foodstuffs including beans, dairy, poultry, cereal grains, and many fruits and vegetables.

While these substances have been banned by both United States law and the Stockholm Convention treaty, (which was independently signed by each of the individual member nations of Codex including the U.S.A.), the Codex Commission itself seems to have little concern about the rampant proliferation of these chemicals in animal feed and byproducts.

Did You Know?

The higher an organism is found in the food chain, the greater amount of POP's can be detected in that organism's body.

Example: *DDT (Dichloro-Diphenyl-Trichloroethane), the first modern toxic chemical pesticide, washes off the land into a lake after a rainstorm. The fish in that lake drink the polluted water, causing DDT to be stored in their body tissues. DDT is not excreted efficiently, and stays in the bodies of fish for a long time—this biomagnifies the chemical (increasing the amount stored in tissues). And guess what? When humans eat fish from that lake, the DDT biomagnifies again! This means that people eating fish contaminated by DDT are actually consuming an exponentially greater amount of the toxic chemical than was originally washed into the lake!*

Shocking Fact: Some studies estimate 99% of the breastmilk in women residing in the United States contains measurable levels of DDT.

One commonly used POP, organochlorine, may also be responsible for contaminating the world's seafood supply, since pesticides can run off from the land into bodies of water. Organochlorines collect in fatty tissue

> **DEFINITION**
>
> ***Essential Fatty Acids:*** Often referred to as Omega-3 and Omega-6 acids, these essential chemicals must be obtained through the diet as the human body cannot manufacture or replicate them.

and remain in an organism for a long time. Fatty fish (such as mackerel, salmon, or tuna), normally a great source of **essential fatty acids**, are fast becoming unsafe to eat in regular quantities.

Because organochlorines break down slowly, they have a tendency to deposit toxic residue in the body over an extended period of time. These harmful chemicals leak through the intestinal lining, accumulate in the body, and can cause headaches, seizures, skin irritation, tremors, respiratory problems, dizziness, and nausea. What's more, many chronic conditions such as cancer, Parkinson's disease, neurological damage, and abnormal immune system function have been linked to organochlorine exposure.

> **DOCTOR'S NOTE:**
>
> *Published U.S. Government studies on the connection between pesticides and cancer have led researchers to investigate the specific connection between organochlorines and colon cancer.*

Had enough red flags by now? Well, let's talk about some solutions to these concerns. Following the tips in the chart below will greatly reduce the number of pesticides in your environment!

How to Eliminate Toxins from Pesticides

- You can reduce the levels of pesticides you consume by 90% just by avoiding the crop items containing the highest levels of pesticide residue. These items include fruits such as peaches, apples, nectarines, strawberries, cherries, pears, grapes, and vegetables such as sweet bell peppers, celery, carrots, and spinach. Of course, if these items are grown organically, they will be okay.

- If you are able, grow your own food using organic growing methods. This is the best way to ensure you are not exposing yourself or your family to pesticides.

- Avoid chemical based mosquito repellents or pesticides in your house or yard. Visit www.organicpesticides.com for natural alternatives.

- By cleansing your intestinal tract with oxygen 2 to 3 times weekly, you can help prevent the accumulation of these cancer-causing agents in your bloodstream.

For a full list of pesticide containing foods, visit www.ewg.org

Will Washing and Peeling Help Reduce Pesticides?

You should always thoroughly wash fresh produce before eating it, but doing so doesn't guarantee you will be able to completely eliminate all the toxic pesticides. The same applies for peeling—it can help reduce the amount of toxins to which your body is exposed, but even this doesn't make food 100% safe. Also, the skin stores a large percentage of the nutrients in many fruits, so peeling them to eat just the interior portion greatly reduces their nutritional value.

How Do Meat and Dairy Cause a Toxic Colon?

If left alone in their natural state, meat and milk are not necessarily bad. However, think about all of the changes meat and dairy products go through before they reach your kitchen. When toxic hormones and antibiotics are injected into animals, they can be passed on to humans,

> **DEFINITION**
>
> *Fodder:*
> Feed (composed mostly of hay and straw) intended for cattle and horses.

thus causing multiple health problems. Also, some studies have suggested that eating as little as three ounces of red meat a day could tip the balance in favor of your developing colon cancer. Naturally occurring live enzymes in milk, on the other hand, are eliminated by the pasteurization process, leaving behind nothing but a "dead" beverage with little to offer. Since the milk is pasteurized, very little if any of the calcium can be absorbed by the body.

➕ DOCTOR'S NOTE:

People who eat just a hamburger's worth of red meat a day are 30 to 40 percent more likely to develop colon cancer than people who eat less than half that amount. Long-term consumption of three or more ounces of processed or "mystery" meat a day (such as hot dogs) increased the risk of developing colon cancer by a whopping 50 percent!

Hormones are naturally occurring chemical messengers produced by all plant and animal species to regulate growth. Synthetic hormone technology is applied to cattle farming to increase meat content and milk production. According to the Sierra Club of Canada, "Hormones are widely used in US agriculture: over 90% of US cattle producers use hormone implants or add them to feed [termed **fodder**]. These hormones are normally administered in a slow-release lozenge-type tablet which is inserted under the cow's skin on their ear. The ears are then cut off and thrown away at slaughter."[16]

Concern is now growing that treated cattle are excreting toxic manure with dangerously high amounts of these hormones. This tainted waste is putting wildlife, the natural environment, and humans at risk.

>
>
> ### Did You Know?
>
> *We normally associate the use of hormones with humans or livestock farming, but even plants are now receiving synthetic or genetically engineered hormones. Cycocel®[17] is a synthetic hormone applied*

> to wheat to produce thicker and longer stems. Researchers are also looking into manipulating the wheat's natural hormones to control germination and also to produce plants that can withstand cold weather.

In addition to being pumped full of hormones, a large percentage of cows are given massive amounts of antibiotics to counteract the rampant infections to which they are vulnerable because of their close-proximity confinement. Even worse—calves are routinely fed the blood of slaughtered cows and other slaughterhouse waste (as "pro-

Milk ... Is It Really So Good?

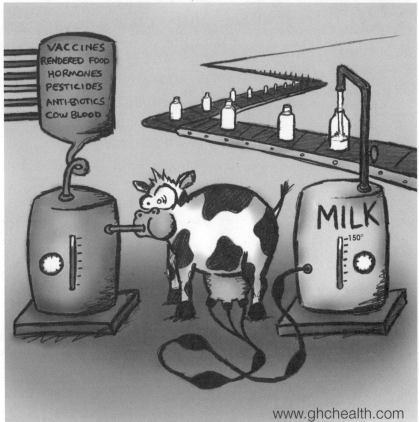

Fig. I

tein") to further boost their hormone and pharmaceutical-induced growth! Robert Cohen, author of *Milk A-Z*, believes, "Ten million tons of blood and entrails, bones, and vital organs ... ground intestinal worms and cancerous tumors ... and the grossest imaginable byproducts of animal slaughter ..." would have to be disposed of annually if this waste were not fed back to cattle, pigs, and chickens.[18]

Where do you think all of these toxic hormones and antibiotics wind up? These toxins collect in the fat, muscle tissue (meat), and milk of the cows and from there to the bodies of consumers. *Cancer Epidemiology, Biomarkers & Prevention* published a British survey concluding the risk of colorectal cancer is increased by up to 20% for each additional portion (approximately 4 ounces) of red meat consumed each week![19]

Shocking Facts About Livestock Farming

- In the United States alone, about 41 million cows are raised and slaughtered for human consumption each year.[20]

- For every pound of beef you eat, factory farmers must use 2,500 gallons of water and a gallon of gasoline to run machinery, and 35 pounds of topsoil is lost due to erosion.[21] As long as we continue to eat meat, we contribute to the loss of our environment.

- Over 1 million animals are slaughtered for human consumption every hour.[22]

- A large portion of U.S. commercial milk cows receive a protein hormone such as bovine growth hormone (rBGH) to increase their milk supply, which has been artificially increased by a factor of 25 in some instances![23]

- Women who consume meat experience a 35% decrease in bone density by the time they reach age 65.[24]

- In the United States, eight times more antibiotics are used for the livestock industry than for human inoculation against disease.[25]

Consuming animal meats and/or processed milk means consuming the accompanying hormones which can alter the human **endocrine system.** The average shoe size of American children has increased in recent years. Women are developing breasts and starting their menstrual cycles at very early ages, primarily due to the combination of growth hormones, testosterone, and estrogen ingested through meat, milk, and cheese products.

> **DEFINITION**
>
> *Endocrine System:* The system of glands regulating bodily processes, including the Hypothalamus, Pineal, Pituitary, Thyroid, Parathyroid, and Adrenal glands.

Surprisingly, women that drink milk have also increased their likelihood of having twins! The likely culprits are insulin-like growth factors (IGF's), a family of proteins found in cow livers that sensitize ovaries and increase egg production when stimulated by a synthetic hormone called recombinant bovine somatotropin (RBS).

➕ DOCTOR'S NOTE:
Cow's milk has been linked to numerous negative health conditions such as allergies, anemia, arthritis, asthma, colic, diabetes, heart disease, Irritable Bowel Syndrome, osteoporosis, stomach ulcers, sinusitis, and a host of infectious and autoimmune diseases. However, current research on organic (unprocessed) raw cow and goat's milk shows are a safer, healthier option.

Yet another toxin lurking in the meat supply is nitrate, which is used to process and cure meats such as bacon, pepperoni, and hot dogs. Nitrates aren't actually cancer-causing agents until they're in the body where they're converted to nitrites. Nitrites are extremely carcinogenic and can increase your risk of developing colon polyps (which, if they become malignant, can lead to cancer). Studies have found that eating processed meat could make you 1.5 to 2 times more likely to develop colorectal polyps and/or cancer.[26]

We've established that meat and dairy products can include hormones, antibiotics, and nitrates, but an even more shocking source of toxins is what is known as "rendered" food materials. Rendered food is what most people unknowingly feed to their pets; but it's also fed to livestock, so it winds up in your local supermarket and then inside your body. We must trace toxins to their root source if we are to eliminate them. What are the animals eating before we eat them? Ultimately, what the animal eats and the environment the animal is exposed to will determine the quality of the meat or dairy derived from them.

In 1990, the *Earth Island Journal* published the best description of rendered food I've ever encountered. The author, who chose to remain anonymous for his own safety and that of his family, sheds light on the inner workings of a feed rendering plant in an article titled "The Dark Side of Recycling."

Warning: *The following excerpt is very graphic!* You may want to skip the next few paragraphs if you think you might be disturbed by such content. I feel it's necessary to share this information with you so you know what really takes place to produce the so-called "nutritious" food you feed to your pets or the animals you eat.

> "The rendering plant floor is piled high with 'raw product.' Thousands of dead dogs and cats, heads and hooves from cattle, sheep, pigs and horses, whole skunks, rats and raccoons—all waiting to be processed. In the 90-degree heat, the piles of dead animals seem to have a life of their own as millions of maggots swarm over the carcasses …
>
> Rendering is the process of cooking raw animal material to remove the moisture and fat. The rendering plant works like a giant kitchen. The cooker, or 'chef', blends the raw product to maintain a certain ratio between the carcasses of pets, livestock, poultry waste, and supermarket rejects …
>
> As the *American Journal of Veterinary Research* explains, this recycled meat and bone meal is used as '… a source of protein and other nutrients in the diets of poultry and swine and in pet foods, with lesser amounts used in the feed of cattle and sheep. Animal fat is also used in animal feeds as an energy source' …
>
> Every day, hundreds of rendering plants in Mexico and across the United States truck millions of tons of this [contaminated] food en-

hancer to poultry ranches, cattle feed-lots, dairy and hog farms, fish-feed plants and pet-food manufacturers where it is mixed with other waste ingredients to feed the billions of animals that meat-eating humans, in turn, will eat ...

> **DEFINITION**
>
> *Euthanasia:*
> A method or technique for killing an animal intended to be humane or relatively pain-free. Lethal injection is a common method for putting an animal "to sleep" or "putting them down."

Rendering plants perform one of the most valuable functions on Earth: they recycle used animals. Without rendering, our cities would run the risk of becoming filled with diseased and rotting carcasses. Fatal viruses, parasites and bacteria would spread uncontrolled through the population. Death is the number one commodity in a business where the demand for feed ingredients far exceeds the supply of raw product. But this elaborate system of food production through waste management has evolved into a recycling nightmare. Rendering plants are unavoidably processing toxic waste...

[As you read, the meat you reject from your store shelf may be "recycled" into this rendering slop and fed to other animals. That's right—the food you rejected because it was spoiled (or just looked bad) might eventually wind up on your plate anyway! On top of that, we're basically forcing our livestock and pets to become cannibals by feeding them rendered animal products that can contain everything from their own species to a variety of organs and roadkill.]

Because [dead] animals are frequently shoved into the pit with flea collars still attached, organophosphate-containing insecticides get into the mix as well. Pharmaceuticals leak from the antibiotics [given to the] livestock, and **[euthanasia]** drugs given to pets are also included. [Think about this the next time your veterinarian says they can "dispose of" your deceased four-legged friend for you. Heavy metals accumulated from a variety of sources such as pet ID tags, surgical pins, needles and even plastics wind up in this supposedly healthy feed ...

Unsold supermarket meats, chicken, and fish arrive in Styrofoam trays and shrink-wrap.] Every week, millions of packages of plastic-wrapped meat go through the rendering process and become one of the unwanted ingredients in animal feed. [Do you think the corporate owners at the processing plants are going to spend money (as hourly wages) on the tedious task of unwrapping thousands of spoiled and rejected meat packs or removing hundreds of flea collars from stray cats and dogs?] More plastic is added to the pits with the inclusion of cattle ID tags, plastic insecticide patches and the [body bags] containing [deceased] pets from veterinarians …

The dead animals (the 'raw') are accompanied by a whole menu of unwanted ingredients. [Pesticides, insecticides, hormones, steroids, euthanasia drugs, and a host of other toxic compounds] enter the rendering process via poisoned livestock, and fish oil laced with bootleg DDT and other organophosphates that have accumulated in the bodies of West Coast mackerel and tuna … Skyrocketing labor costs are one of the economic factors forcing the corporate flesh-peddlers to cheat. It is far too costly for plant personnel to cut off flea collars or unwrap, spoiled T-bone steaks. Every week, millions of packages of plastic-wrapped spoiled meat go through the rendering process and become one of the unwanted ingredients in animal feed."[27]

Still Want That Supermarket Steak?

On the following page are my suggestions for saving our animals and eliminating these toxins from your daily diet.

How to Eliminate Toxins from Meat and Dairy

- Eat hormone and antibiotic-free, range-fed, organic meats or wild game. Buffalo and ostrich meat are healthful alternatives to beef.

- Limit meat intake to 1 to 3 meals weekly, if necessary.

- Eat more fish but make sure it's free of pesticides and mercury. For details about mercury contamination in fish, see *Chapter 10—How to Eliminate Intestinal Toxins from Heavy Metals and Radiation*.

- Avoid processed meat at all costs! This includes bacon, hot dogs, sandwich meat, etc.

- Replace cow's milk with hemp milk, rice milk, almond milk, or raw goat's milk. Better yet, drink only purified water! My personal favorite is hemp milk. It is delicious with a slightly nutty flavor and provides essential and balanced nutrition. Hemp milk is a fantastic alternative to soymilk or cows' milk. For an easy recipe, see the *Resources* section.

- Consume only organic cheese or goat cheese.

- Whenever you eat meat, take an enzyme supplement to assist your body with proper digestion.

- Chew each bite of food 25 times before swallowing to reduce the burden on your stomach and intestines.

- Eat more vegetables and smaller portions of meat during each meal.

How to Eliminate Toxins from Meat and Dairy (contd.)

- Test your stomach acid levels. If they are low, begin supplementing with a beet-derived HCl (hydrochloric acid) substitute. A natural healthcare practitioner can likely provide this.

For more information about healthy foods, see *Chapter 6—The Colon Diet*.

How Does Soy Cause a Toxic Colon?

The reported health benefits and marketing of soy-based food products have led to significantly increased popularity worldwide. Soy marketers advertise benefits covering everything from heart disease to menopause, but is soy really nature's "miracle food", or is its reputation just a bunch of hype?

A frequently heard argument is that soy plays a key role in the long, healthy lifespan enjoyed by the Japanese people. Why then, is the life expectancy of the average American so much shorter than that of the Japanese if we consume large amounts of soybeans?

Literally tons of products consumed in the United States contain soy, but the bean's popularity in the U.S. is a fairly recent development. Maybe soy just hasn't been part of the American diet long enough to make a noticeable difference. That wouldn't be a bad guess, but it's still wrong. The real difference lies in the fact that the Japanese eat *fermented* soy, which is drastically different from the unfermented soy found in dry soybeans, soymilk, and tofu. Fermented soy products, such as fermented soymilk, tofu, miso, soy sauces, tempeh, and natto, may on the other hand help prevent certain cancers and other diseases.

This may be largely due to the fermentation process increasing the amount of available isoflavones in the soy. Fermentation makes use of live organisms. Unfermented soy products in America are not only deficient in isoflavones, but they are full of natural toxins that can block essential enzymes needed for protein digestion.

Dr. Joseph Mercola notes "Soybeans are high in phytic acid, present in the bran or hulls of all seeds. It's a substance that can block the uptake of essential minerals - calcium, magnesium, copper, iron and especially zinc - in the intestinal tract."[28] He adds that a large percentage of soy is also genetically modified and/or contaminated by pesticides.

How to Eliminate Toxins from Soy

- Do not drink soymilk.

- Never feed your child soy-based infant formulas!

- Avoid eating soy-based products unless they have been fermented. Natto, tempeh, miso, soy sauces, and fermented tofu are all safe options.

- Be weary of soy meat substitutes and items containing hydrolyzed vegetable protein—they're often made from soy.

- Margarine, vegetable oils, shortenings, mayonnaise, and salad dressings are also common places to find soy. Read the labels before buying.

- Be on the lookout for soy when dining at Asian food restaurants. If you are in doubt, always ask whether or not a dish contains soy.

- Read the labels on all food products when you shop. You may be surprised just how many products contain soy. Products containing lecithin, MSG, or "natural flavors"

How to Eliminate Toxins from Soy (contd.)

almost always contain soy. Avoiding processed foods altogether is a good way to help keep hidden soy (and other ingredients) out of your diet.

How Does White Flour Cause a Toxic Colon?

White flour is a common ingredient made from grains of wheat. Unlike whole grain flour, which utilizes wheat in its entirety (starch, protein, and fiber), white flour is made from just the starchy part. In effect, the healthful parts of the wheat are removed. Synthetic B-vitamins engineered from petrochemicals (derived from coal tar), are then added to replace the natural B-vitamins removed, which cause imbalances in the body. These synthetic vitamins are usually labeled thiamine (B1), riboflavin (B2), niacin (B3), and calcium pantothenate (B5).

Did You Know?

In a study where pigs were fed large amounts of synthetic B vitamins, the pigs produced sterile offspring. Synthetic vitamins provide no nutritional value—they are poisonous!

Since white flour contains no fiber, it is difficult to pass through the large intestine. Processed foods often contain large amounts of white flour that can cause constipation and significantly increase waste transit time, and this gives toxins more time to enter the bloodstream.

If that isn't bad enough, white flour is often bleached to get rid of its freshly milled yellow color and to increase the amount of gluten the flour can produce. Chlorine, acetone peroxide, benzoyl peroxide, and nitrogen dioxide are the most common oxidizing agents used during white flour processing.

Did You Know?

The average American colon processes approximately 200 pounds of white flour each year.

People who regularly eat white bread, white rice, and processed potatoes are at increased risk for developing diabetes, but these foods can be easily replaced with whole grain alternatives. Carefully check labels when you are at the grocery store. Many products marketed as being made with "whole grains" are actually made from white flour and contain just a small amount of the original substance.

How to Eliminate Toxins from White Flour

- Avoid foods made with white or "enriched" flour. Enriched flour is bad for you because the nutrients have been replaced with derivatives of coal tar.

- Replace white breads and pasta with whole grains or sprouted grain flour. You can purchase whole grain products online or purchase them from natural food markets. Whole grains should be soaked or sprouted to avoid irritation to the intestinal lining.

- Start by reducing your white flour intake to just 2 times weekly.

- Regular colon cleansing (2 to 3 times weekly) can help relieve

> ### How to Eliminate Toxins from White Flour (contd.)
>
> symptoms of constipation and toxin buildup associated with eating white flour.
>
> - Avoid foods commonly made from white flour: breads (even those labeled as "multigrain" or "wheat"), pizza crusts, pasta, bagels, pretzels, crackers, tortillas, hamburger and hot dog buns, and most breakfast cereals.

How Does Table Salt Cause a Toxic Colon?

The Center for Science in the Public Interest, a nutritional lobbying group, claims that sodium chloride (common table salt) could be "… the single deadliest ingredient in the food supply."[29] The CSPI has recommended to the FDA to change the status of salt from "generally recognized as safe" (which leaves it essentially unregulated), to "food additive" since this would give the FDA more authority to regulate its use in foods.

The idea of regulating table salt may sound ridiculous at first but it's actually a great idea. Remember the Japanese and their long lifespans? Well, it seems there's always a catch. Many of the fermented soy products the Japanese consume are overloaded with refined table salt. In fact, much research suggests "…dietary factors, especially sodium … are of primary importance as determinants of stroke mortality."[30] Also, the abnormally high incidence of stomach cancer in certain Asian countries (such as Korea) may be related to the quantity of salt in the diet.

Two types of salt exist—good salt (living) and bad salt (dead and refined). Salt is a natural antibiotic—meaning, it kills life! That's why salt has been used as a preservative for thousands of years. By killing bacterial life in a food, salt is able to slow the natural decomposition of that food. Salt also draws water from the bloodstream, causing the body to experience excessive thirst. These two factors above all others contribute to salt's damaging effects on the digestive system.

Refined salt's antibiotic properties reduce the beneficial bacteria that normally aid the digestive tract in processing waste. Simultaneously, salt's dehydrating effects interfere with the absorption of water, which leads to possible constipation and the accumulation of toxins.

Most packaged, canned, and restaurant foods contain large amounts of refined table salt. Fortunately, the popularity of low-sodium diets has led many companies to offer reduced-salt options. Be careful however, a large discrepancy exists between the terms "less sodium," "low sodium," and the real meaning of low sodium. Most table salt is depleted of vital minerals and contains harmful additives such as aluminum-silicate or corn sugar (both of which are toxic to the body) to prevent it from clumping.

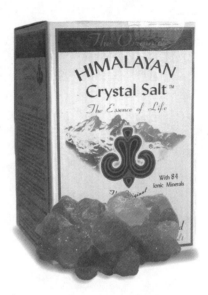

Fig. II: Himalayan Crystal Salt

Natural salts (such as "sea salt") are now being marketed as a replacement to table salt but most of these salts are also partially refined. On the other hand, Himalayan Salt or Celtic Sea Salt are living substances, produced with ancient drying methods, and contain the vital minerals we need. Our body fluids closely resemble the structure of seawater, so these salts are quite beneficial for balancing internal fluids. I personally recommend Himalayan Crystal Salt™ because it contains all the elements and minerals your body needs without any of the toxins found in common table salt.

Health Benefits of Himalayan Salt

- Balances blood sugar and acid levels and helps the body's cells generate electrical energy
- Acts as a natural antihistamine by regulating phlegm and mucus in the sinuses and nasal cavity
- Helps prevent osteoporosis, muscle cramping, and irregular heartbeat
- Promotes healthy sleep and intimacy patterns

How to Eliminate Toxins from Table Salt

- Replace table salt with natural Himalayan salt or Celtic Sea Salt. These are natural (not processed by humans).

- Try using Braggs™ Liquid Aminos to flavor dishes you would normally salt. This product is rich in essential and non-essential amino acids and flavors meals well.

- When you are dining out, try ordering fresh foods or order homemade foods and specifically request No Salt!

- For extra flavor, try using fresh herbs, or lemon or lime juice instead of table salt.

- Cleanse your colon regularly to prevent constipation caused by table salt's dehydrating effects.

See the *Resources* section at the end of this book for additional product and purchasing information.

How Does Monosodium Glutamate (MSG) Cause a Toxic Colon?

Glutamate is a naturally occurring amino acid found in foods that contain protein, such as milk, mushrooms, and fish. MSG (monosodium glutamate) is a manufactured flavor-enhancing food additive comprised of just the sodium salt of glutamate. MSG is widely distributed in the food industry, and is most often disguised with deceptive product labels used to hide its presence.

Avoid the Following Products or Ingredients Containing MSG

- Autolyzed yeast
- Bouillon broth
- Calcium Caseinate
- Corn oil
- Cosmetics
- Foods with labels advertising "no added MSG"
- Frozen and canned foods
- Hydrolyzed oat flour
- Hydrolyzed vegetable protein
- Infant formulas
- Malt extract
- Malt flavoring
- Natural flavors/flavoring
- Plant protein extract
- Restaurant foods
- Seasoning
- Some dietary supplements
- Sodium Caseinate
- Spices
- Stock flavoring
- Textured protein
- Vaccines
- Wine
- Yeast extract

According to the national consumer watchdog group, Truthinlabeling.org:

> "The distinction between having MSG poured into an ingredient and processed into an ingredient is important because the glutamate industry plays on this distinction in their efforts to hide the presence of MSG. One of their favorite ways of hiding MSG is to claim that there is "no added MSG" in a product. If MSG is processed into a product instead of being poured into a product, they declare that there is "no MSG added" or "no added MSG," in the product, even though they know the product contains MSG. The glutamate industry is adamantly opposed to letting consumers know where MSG

is hidden. Why? Because the glutamate industry is fully aware that MSG is a toxic substance and causes adverse reactions, brain lesions, endocrine disorders, and other negative health problems."[31]

DOCTOR'S NOTE:

Since MSG was introduced into the American diet, the incidence of Type II Diabetes has doubled in the past 30 years in the U.S. Obesity rates in children have also skyrocketed. MSG is also injected in laboratory animals to induce obesity for testing various pharmaceutical drugs. So, if you have a weight problem, it may be associated with hidden MSG intake.

Serious health conditions have been reported following the consumption of even trace amounts of MSG. These problems range from asthma, headaches, skin irritations, gastrointestinal disturbances, allergies, obesity, diabetes, adrenal gland malfunction, seizures, high blood pressure, hypothyroidism, stroke, and heart complications. If you are experiencing any of those conditions, it is imperative to eliminate MSG from your diet immediately.

How to Eliminate Toxins from MSG

- Read all food labels at the supermarket. Avoid products containing MSG.

- Always ask if the restaurant's dishes contain MSG when dining out.

- Stay away from fast food! Most of these establishments use MSG in their fries and drinks to make them taste better and get you addicted to their foods.

- Cleanse your colon regularly to prevent the swelling of the mucus membranes in the gastrointestinal tract caused by consumption of MSG.

Now you know how to avoid the most damaging intestinal toxins from food, but you still need to learn how to prepare fresh, delicious, organic food. For example, should you eat organic foods as a raw salad or lightly cook them for a few minutes along with a pasta dish? Does it really matter? Absolutely!

> **DEFINITION**
>
> ***Anti-catarrhal Factors:*** Any substance which aids in removing mucous and reducing inflammation of the mucous membranes.

Cooking Food the Wrong Way!

"I'd like the grilled chicken breast with sautéed vegetables, please." Most people would be proud of themselves for ordering that dish instead of a hamburger and fries. Unfortunately, it's not as healthful as you might think. As the vegetables are heated, precious enzymes and vitamins can be reduced or destroyed; they are no longer living sources of energy. Charles de Coti-Marsh stated a balanced uncooked meal, "...provides all the vitamins for the body's defense against diseases, **anti-catarrhal factors,** anti-ageing factors, anti-arthritic factors, anti-excess-calcium factors, sunshine vitamins, anti-sterility factors and rebuilding factors."[32]

Let's consider the nutritious value of that seemingly healthy order of grilled chicken. Grilling meats (as well as barbecuing and broiling them) can produce HCA's (heterocyclic-amines) which are known cancer-causing agents. Seventeen different HCA's have been identified as byproducts of cooking meats at high temperatures. A connection also exists between fried or baked starches and the formation of carcinogens.

Mark Kaufman [In an article for the Washington Post] addresses the findings of a Swedish study: "The chemical, acrylamide, which is used industrially in the manufacturing of some plastics, is also apparently formed by the heating of starches. Foods with especially high levels of the chemical included French fries, potato chips and crackers."[33]

What About Cooking Food in a Microwave Oven?

Let's say you want to heat up last night's macaroni and cheese in the microwave for a minute or two. When you take it out of the microwave, it might still look, smell, and taste like macaroni and cheese, but what you have is essentially a radiated pile of zero-nutrient garbage.

The microwave radiation causes water, fat, and sugar molecules to rotate very quickly to create friction and this is what generates the heat to cook the food from the inside out. This sounds convenient, but the radiation also destroys the chemical bonds giving these compounds their nutritional value.

According to Anthony Wayne and Lawrence Newell of the Christian Law Institute & Fellowship Assembly, "Radiation causes ionization, which is what occurs when a neutral atom gains or loses electrons. In simpler terms, a microwave oven decays and changes the molecular structure of the food by the process of radiation."[34] The radiation breaks down any vitamins and minerals in the food and changes their natural

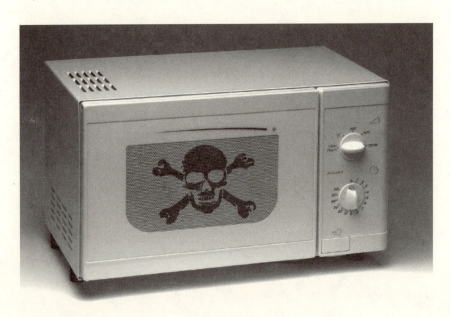

structure. Your body cannot handle these irradiated molecules and they eventually weaken your immune and digestive system from the harmful molecules and the lack of proper nutrition.

Important Facts about the Toxic Effects of Microwaves

1. Drs. Hans Ulrich Hertel and Dr. Bernard H. Blanc performed a clinical study, which first appeared in the journal *Franz Weber*, showing the degenerative forces of microwave ovens. It was concluded that microwave cooking changed the nutrients in the food, leading to changes in the consumer's blood that could damage bodily systems.

2. In the December 9, 1989 *Lancet*, Dr. Lita Lee reported that microwave warming of some baby formulas transforms certain trans-amino acids into synthetic substances such as trans-fats. L-Proline, one of the amino acids, converts to a poisonous substance that harms the kidneys and the nervous system.

3. The Soviet Union banned microwaves in 1976 and issued a worldwide health warning based on research that began in the 1950s. The research suggests that people who consume microwave-cooked food are more likely to develop stomach and intestinal cancers, peripheral cellular tissue degeneration, and a gradual breakdown of the digestive and excretory system.

4. In an article published by *Perceptions* in 1996 entitled "Microwave Madness: The effects of Microwave Apparatus on Food and Humans", the authors (Kopp and William) state stomach and intestinal cancer is especially high in people who eat microwaved foods.

For the sake of your health, I want you to walk into your kitchen, unplug your microwave (if you have one), and get rid of it! Heating food in a microwave is called "nuking" for a good reason. Irradiated food is dead before you even eat it. Remember—your body wants to live and it needs foods that are high in energy not toxins.

How to Eliminate Toxins from Microwaved Food and Drinks

- Ask all restaurants if they use a microwave to reheat or cook foods. If so, request that your food be steamed, grilled on the range, or broiled or baked in the oven.

- Replace your microwave with an air-convection oven.

- Cook the old-fashioned way. Use non-toxic cookware. I recommend glass, terracotta (without lead glaze), titanium, silicone, or cast iron cookware. Avoid aluminum, Teflon®-coated, copper, and stainless steel (inferior grades contain Nickel to reduce costs) cookware.[35]

- Avoid heating beverages such as water and coffee in the microwave.

After looking at the evidence of toxicity involved in modern food processing, production, and preparation, you may be thinking it's a lost cause trying to eat healthy. It's not, though. You can control the amount of toxins you ingest from food by applying positive changes to your daily habits. You don't have to put all of my suggestions in place today. Getting your digestive system on the right track won't occur overnight. Just focusing on a few changes at a time can increase your body's energy levels and improve your overall health.

Eliminating Intestinal Toxins from Beverages

Unfortunately, many of the beverages we enjoy create a highly toxic environment within the digestive tract. Think about a can of soda–it doesn't have just one source of toxins but several! First, the acids used to flavor or carbonate colas can irritate the sensitive intestinal lining. Second, the sweet taste of the soda is either due to the addition of refined sugar (bad) or a sugar substitute (very bad).

Third, if your soda is caffeinated, it is also toxic to the gastrointestinal tract. Coffee, another caffeinated drink which many people have come to depend on daily, can be especially damaging to the bowels. Coffee also disrupts the growth of healthy digestive flora. Alcoholic beverages are also dangerous sources of colon toxins. Let me show you just how addictive these beverages (or legal drugs I say) really can be in your body.

A Drug Addiction Story

Instead of going to a drug dealer, a young child gets his drug from his parents, friends, and his school multiple times every day. He is innocent and does not even realize he has a tragic addiction to a powerful drug. This drug is not only legal; it is freely available to him almost anytime he craves it. This boy has been addicted to this drug since early childhood and suffers daily from the side effects of depression, attention deficit, acne, weight fluctuations, lack of self-confidence and self-esteem, fatigue, constipation, and anxiety—and yet he's only a child.

The boy continues to cry out for help, but no one listens. When he comes home from school, he has access to even more of the drug in his home. His parents and school teachers continue teaching him not to do drugs, not to smoke, not to drink alcohol, yet they are feeding his addiction with one of the most toxic

> drugs of all time!
>
> Believe it or not—the "drug" in question is a common soft drink or energy drink perceived by most people as just another beverage. By age 14 (or even sooner), he is overweight and newly diagnosed with diabetes and a slew of other health problems.
>
> He is ultimately prescribed daily insulin shots and other toxic pharmaceutical drugs as a "cure" while his life slowly begins to deteriorate. He continues this decline throughout his life until both of his feet are amputated as the final "treatment" for his diabetes. And to make matters worse, since childhood he was provided this DRUG by the people who loved him the most!

Although this is a harsh and sad story, it happens all too often. The worst part is—parents are not even taking the time to research and protect their children from these deadly drugs because they have also been addicted since early childhood and so the cycle continues. Everyone thinks, "It's okay. What's the harm of a soda now and then? You gotta' live a little right?" But when does "living" involve a lifetime of poor health?

Nevertheless, you can make change happen! If we all start working together, we can change the world one day at a time. Just by eliminating half of your daily soda intake, you can make great strides towards beating the sugar addiction. On a personal note, I just experienced the wonderful birth of my first son and I swear I will never put him through the kind of misery described above. My son is being taught to avoid these poisons and raised without toxin-filled junk foods in his diet.

Regardless of how you may feel about them, sodas are addictive and they are a type of drug. It does not matter what kind of soda or brand you think about—at least one verifiably toxic ingredient was used in its synthesis.

How Does Refined Sugar Cause a Toxic Colon?

In 1998, the Center for Science in the Public Interest (CSPI) published a report called *Liquid Candy*. This report states, "Companies annually produce enough soda to provide 557 12-ounce cans ... to every man, woman, and child ... Carbonated drinks are the single biggest source of refined sugars in the American diet ... providing the average 12- to 19-year-old boy with about 15 teaspoons of refined sugars a day."[36] Keep in mind that's just an average from nearly ten years ago. Today, a 12-ounce soft drink or "energy drink" often contains 8 or more teaspoons of sugar in a single can! Commercial fruit juices can be just as bad. Many of them contain only 10 percent or less real fruit juice. Guess where the rest of the flavor is coming from—refined sugar and artificial flavorings.

Did You Know?

- *It's estimated the average American colon processes approximately 100 pounds of refined sugar and 75 pounds of high fructose corn syrup every year.*

- *Dentists are reporting that the front teeth of many young boys and girls are almost completely void of enamel from drinking too much soda. "One-fifth of one- and two-year-old children consume soft drinks ..." so please reconsider how damaging it is to put a little soda in your child's bottle or sippy-cup.*[37]

- *"In 2004, Americans spent $66 billion on carbonated drinks—and billions more on noncarbonated soft drinks. That works out to about $850 per household—enough to buy a computer and year's worth of Internet access."*[38]

- *In 2005, carbonated drink sales exceeded 10 billion cases— equaling roughly $69 billion dollars in revenue!*[39]

> - *In 1993, School District 11 in Colorado Springs signed a contract with Coca-Cola®. The soft drink giant "...Coca-Cola generates millions of dollars for [the district in exchange for] ... signage rights to school buses, public address announcements at each varsity basketball and football game, a full-page ad in football athletic programs, logo inclusion on the district's website, twenty all-sports season tickets, ads in three issues of the district's newsletter and more."*
>
> *According to the contract, school administrators were required to encourage students to drink sodas (even in class) to meet annual sales quotas and "... Coke machines were placed in locker rooms, and athletic directors emptied them each week and used the change to purchase equipment."[40] Since when do colas improve athletic performance? Obviously, achievement was outweighed by profit in School District 11. Although many schools are now making efforts to remove junk food from their campuses, parents and caregivers must be constantly vigilant for such self-supporting actions taken by school educators and administrators.*

Reading the labels of sweet snacks and drinks can be confusing and manufacturers will often mask sugar as something else. Don't let the following terms fool you—they're all variants of refined sugar.

Refined Sugar May Appear on the Label As ...

- Amazake
- Carob powder
- Corn Syrup
- Dextrose
- High fructose corn syrup
- Maple syrup
- Molasses
- Processed Fructose
- Sorbitol
- Sucrose
- Turbinado
- White Sugar

DID YOU KNOW... ONE OF THE MANY STEPS FOR REFINING SUGAR INCLUDES BLEACHING (TO OBTAIN THAT "PURE" WHITE COLOR) WITH ANIMAL CHARCOAL FROM DEGREASED COW BONES?

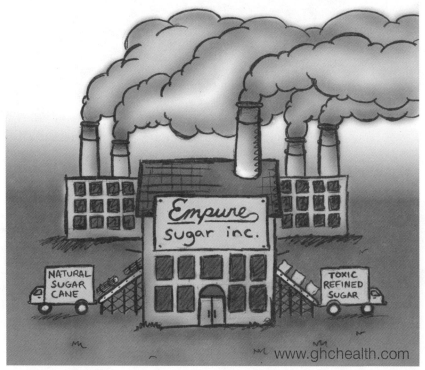

Fig. III

In 1957, Dr. William Coda Martin offered the following definition of a poison. "Medically: Any substance applied to the body, ingested or developed within the body, which causes or may cause disease. Physically: Any substance which inhibits the activity of a catalyst which is a minor substance, chemical or enzyme that activates a reaction."[41] Dr. Martin classified refined sugar as a poison because it is depleted of its life force, vitamins, and minerals.

Sugar ingested daily produces a continuously altered internal pH, meaning the body becomes more acidic. More minerals are drawn from deep within the body in an attempt to restore a proper balance. For example, to protect the blood, calcium is taken from the bones and teeth in such great amounts that decay and weakening of the bones begins and this leads to osteoarthritis. Consumption of refined sugar can damage the digestive tract and eventually affect every organ in the body.

How to Eliminate Toxins from Refined Sugar

- Replace refined sugars with organic agave nectar, xylitol, raw cane sugar, or locally grown unprocessed honey.

- Eliminate soft drinks from your daily routine. Eliminate 12 ounces (1 can) daily until you kick the habit completely.

- Avoid "energy drinks" and store bought "fruit flavored" juices made from concentrate.

- Limit sweets to no more than 3 times weekly and buy all-natural or organic sweets containing natural sugars.

- When you have a craving for sweets or soda, eat fresh fruit such as watermelon or citrus fruits instead. This will help stabilize your blood sugar and satisfy the body's craving for sugar.

- Cleanse your colon 2 to 3 times weekly with a high quality oxygen based colon cleanser to reduce the acidic environment in the bowel and also the excessive fermentation of sugars.

- Try mixing equal parts fresh fruit juice and club soda to create your own delicious soft drinks and punches.

- Drink unsweetened herbal tea with lemon, lime, or fresh mint to add flavor.

- Instead of sugary drinks, drink purified water as often as possible!

Colon Toxins from Artificial Sweeteners

> **DEFINITION**
>
> *Carcinogen:* Any chemical, material, or other foreign substance known to cause cancer.

Artificial sweeteners are food additives that mimic the flavor of sugar but contain virtually no useful energy. In the United States, the following five sugar substitutes are approved for consumer use: saccharin, neotame, acesulfame potassium, aspartame, and sucralose. We will focus on sucralose and aspartame as two of the most widespread and dangerous artificial sweeteners.

Sucralose, a fairly new artificial sweetener, can already be found in a wide variety of products including beverages and baking goods. Surprisingly, some nutritionally oriented companies manufacture products containing sucralose and health stores actually carry them, but is sucralose proven safe? Does sucralose provide any benefit (such as aiding in weight loss) to the public? Is this sweetener safe for the environment? Have any long-term studies been conducted on humans consuming this artificial sugar? Unfortunately, the answer to all of these questions is a resounding no! So why is this product allowed to be manufactured and sold?

Belonging to the supposed "next generation" of high-intensity sugar substitutes, sucralose is most recognized and sold under the name Splenda®.[42] Sucralose is a non-caloric, white crystalline powder that tastes a lot like sugar but is much sweeter. Sucralose is about 600 times sweeter than sucrose (refined table sugar) but it can range from 320 to 1,000 times sweeter depending on the food or beverage containing it. Sucralose is produced by chlorinating sucrose. This involves chemically changing the structure of the sugar molecules by substituting three chlorine atoms for three hydroxyl groups. The changes caused by chlorination raise a big red flag in my opinion. Chlorine is a known **carcinogen**, so why is the FDA allowing something toxic to be included in our food and beverages?

Reasons to Avoid Sucralose

The Holistic Healing Web Page cites the follow reasons to steer clear of sucralose:

- Pre-approval research indicated the potential toxicity of sucralose, but the FDA approved it anyway.
- No independent, controlled, or long term human studies exist for sucralose (similar to the Aspartame studies from 15 years ago).
- Neither federal regulators nor consumer watch groups monitor the safety of sucralose.[43]

Without sufficient monitoring, the effects of harmful substances can go largely undetected. Due to a lack of **epidemiological** research, it took decades for government agencies to finally agree there were countless tobacco-related deaths. Without monitoring and research, it is impossible to determine the safety of substances such as sucralose. To help avoid damage to your intestinal lining, avoid all products containing this artificial compound.

What Do I Need to Know About Aspartame?

Aspartame, originally marketed by the Monsanto Chemical Co., is commonly sold by the brand names Equal® or Nutrasweet®.[44] Aspartame is yet another dangerous chemical food additive and is contained in at least 5,000 products around the world. Common products include "diet" carbonated and non-carbonated drinks, yogurt, pudding, tabletop sweeteners (for restaurants), chewing gum, frozen confections, and even vitamins and cough drops.

> **DEFINITION**
> *Epidemiological:* The branch of science concerned with public health and the causes of disease.

NutraSweet® was first produced by G. D. Searle Company. The Searle Company was due to be prosecuted by the U. S. Justice Department for fabricating test results indicating that Aspartame was safe (and later for racketeering charges) but legal matters were held up and delayed by unscrupulous attorneys (whom later took extremely lucrative positions within the Aspartame industry) until the statute of limitations expired. An initial investigation titled "The Bressler Report" details numerous discrepancies between reported study data and the actual, verifiable data describing the toxicity of Aspartame.[45]

Symptoms of Aspartame Poisoning

Aspartame has been linked to at least 92 documented side effects, including:

- Amyotrophic Lateral Sclerosis (Lou Gehrig's Disease)
- Alzheimer's disease
- Anxiety
- Blurred vision
- Cancer
- CFS (Chronic Fatigue Syndrome)
- Cramps
- Depression
- Diabetes
- Diarrhea
- Dizziness
- Headaches
- Heart palpitations or seizures
- Hypertension
- Joint pain
- Memory loss
- Multiple Sclerosis
- Muscle spasms
- Nausea
- Numbness
- PMS
- Rashes
- Sexual dysfunction
- Vertigo
- Vomiting
- Weight gain

In a dramatic article titled *The Aspartame Scandal,* Betty Martini reports, "The FDA has received more than 10,000 consumer complaints on this Nutra-Poison. That's 80% of all complaints about food additives, yet they remain comatose and have done nothing to alert the American consumer who assumes, since it's so highly advertised, that it must be as safe as mother's milk."[46]

As part of her research, Ms. Martini quotes from *Flying Safety*–an official United States Air Force publication stating that pilots were warned not to consume Aspartame in any amounts whatsoever. Aspartame has been investigated as a possible cause of brain tumors, mental retardation, birth defects, epilepsy, Parkinson's Disease, Fibromyalgia, and Diabetes, yet the FDA (that once sought to have Aspartame removed from the market) has done nothing to regulate this toxic artificial sweetener!

Did You Know?

After being inside the body for 20 minutes, Aspartame begins breaking down from its original compound into methanol, formaldehyde (a Class-A carcinogen used to embalm corpses) and formic acid (ant venom).

How to Eliminate Toxins from Artificial Sweeteners

- Go through your pantry and refrigerator and throw out everything that has any of the following artificial sweeteners listed on the label: Aspartame, Acesulfame Potassium (K), Saccharin, or Sucralose.

- Avoid any product claiming to be "low calorie," "diet," "sugar free," or "no added sugar". All of these likely contain artificial sweeteners.

- Replace diet drinks with pure, clean purified water. Water provides zero calories!

- Avoid the following brands: Equal®, Nutrasweet®, and Splenda®.

- Write letters to your political representatives and the FDA asking them to protect your health by banning toxic artificial sweeteners.

- Replace artificial sweeteners with natural sweeteners such as agave nectar, xylitol, or locally grown honey. Use organic sources whenever possible.

- Cleanse your intestinal tract regularly to help reduce and eliminate the toxic effects of artificial sweeteners.

- Cleanse your liver and gallbladder to detoxify your body of built up toxins. See Chapter 12—Dr. Group's Liver, Gallbladder, Parasite Cleanse and Heavy Metal Cleanse.

- For more information on the toxic effects of artificial sweeteners, visit: www.sweetpoison.com

How Does Caffeine Affect My Colon?

Caffeine is a highly addictive compound that many people have come to depend on for the perception of increased energy. Caffeine is found naturally in tea, coffee, and cocoa and is added to many carbonated beverages. Caffeine keeps you going by preventing the chemical adenosine from telling the brain it's time to relax. The result is a surge of unnatural energy; but over time, the brain becomes accustomed to the threshold and requires ever-greater amounts of caffeine to provide the same increase in alertness. This is what makes caffeine products such as coffee so addictive and it explains why the line at Starbucks® is always so long.

"Caffeine's addictiveness, in fact, may be one reason why six of the seven most popular soft drinks contain caffeine," reports the Center for Science in the Public Interest.[47] It's easy to become hooked if you're exposed to caffeinated beverages early on. With the addition of soft drink machines in elementary and junior high schools, and coffee shops on every corner, we are creating a nation of people that are physiologically dependent on this addictive toxin.

Drinking caffeinated beverages can dehydrate the body and interfere with digestion. Caffeine also interferes with the absorption of magnesium, which is critical in maintaining regular, healthy bowel movements.

Coffee over-stimulates the digestive system and can induce a temporary laxative effect, causing the bowels to expel waste before it's had the chance to process and utilize vital water and nutrients. This frequently leads to a constant state of dehydration and malnourishment among coffee drinkers. This effect is not only due to the caffeine in coffee—the same effects are seen in people who regularly drink decaffeinated varieties.

Coffee is also highly acidic and can lead to an overproduction of stomach acid that can severely irritate the intestines. Unbelievably, decaffeinated coffee has been shown to trigger even more acid production than regular coffee. This over-production (when combined with coffee's laxative effects) can cause too much stomach acid to move into the intestines. All this acid can potentially cause irreversible damage to the intestinal lining.

DOCTOR'S NOTE:

Slowly eliminating caffeine from your diet may actually relieve the following conditions: Irritable Bowel Syndrome, acid reflux, stomach ulcers, diarrhea, Crohn's disease, high blood pressure, difficulty sleeping, anxiety, and Ulcerative Colitis.

Did You Know?

Over 70% of the world's coffee supply is contaminated with toxic pesticides and chemicals. It's estimated that just one cup of coffee contains more than 2,000 chemicals, many of which are gastrointestinal irritants and cancer-causing agents. Also, The high heat used in roasting coffee beans causes the natural oils to turn rancid, further contributing to its chemical load.

Kicking the Coffee Habit

Many people think they need coffee just to make it through their daily routine. Overcoming a coffee addiction is one of the best things you can do for colon health. I recommend slowly eliminating coffee from your daily routine. Try substituting store-bought coffee with natural grain coffee. Grain coffee is to coffee as herbal tea is to tea, and grain coffee is naturally caffeine-free. Grain coffee is a ground mixture of grains, nuts, and dried fruit and provides only natural flavors. Grain coffee is available in regular drip coffee-maker and instant brands.

These coffee substitutes come in a variety of flavors: vanilla nut, java, hazelnut, chocolate mint, almond amaretto, etc. A great way to transition to grain coffee is to mix it with regular coffee as you scoop the dry grounds into your coffee filter. So if you normally use 4 scoops of ground coffee, then try 3 scoops of coffee with 1 scoop of grain coffee for the first week. Continue to transition gradually until you have eliminated your consumption of regular coffee altogether.

I don't recommend decaffeinated coffee or tea because known carcinogens are used in the decaffeination process, and decaffeinated drinks are still highly acidic.

Are you addicted to caffeine?
A good way to tell is if you experience withdrawal symptoms such as mood swings, headaches, and/or fatigue whenever you avoid caffeine for a day or two. Don't worry though, this is only temporary and can be greatly reduced by drinking large amounts of water and taking an oxygen-based intestinal cleanser.

How to Eliminate Toxins from Caffeine and Coffee

- Slowly reduce your intake of caffeinated beverages. Replace those beverages with herbal teas or coffee substitutes such as Teeccino®, Pero®, or Roma® brands. (See "Coffee" in the *Resources* section)

- If you must drink coffee, use only organic varieties to help reduce the number of pesticides, fertilizers, and other contaminants from commercial coffee growing techniques.

- Drink plenty of water with raw organic Apple Cider Vinegar to help renew your body and provide you with more energy. You may even find you don't need that "boost" from caffeinated products anymore!

- Clean your colon weekly to prevent irritation and excess acid in the bowel caused by regular coffee consumption.

- Use natural unbleached filters in drip coffee makers to reduce your exposure to bleaching agents.

- If you drink decaffeinated coffee, be aware that most of the major brands use chemicals to decaffeinate their product even when they claim to be "naturally decaffeinated."

- If your children are addicted to caffeine, please help them quit now! Otherwise, they may deal with this drug addiction for the rest of their lives.

How Does Alcohol Cause Colon Toxins?

Alcohol is another one of those readily available beverages posing a serious health risk. It's estimated over 100 million people in the United

States regularly consume alcohol. As a matter of fact, the National Survey on Drug Use and Health (NSDUH) provides data that "...more than half of Americans aged 12 or older reported being current drinkers of alcohol."[48]

More than 6 percent of the same demographic also reported heavy drinking on a regular basis (roughly 5 or more drinks at one time at least 5 days per month).[49] At this rate, it could be said one in twenty consumers possesses a notable drinking problem, yet over 90 percent of this sample felt they did not have a drinking problem![50] Alcoholic beverages disrupt a number of body processes, including those of the liver and gastrointestinal tract, and cause a host of societal and interpersonal problems.

Alarming Statistics about Alcohol Consumption in the United States

- Nearly a third of kids and teens are underage drinkers, regardless if they live in a city or small town.[51]

- The National Institute on Alcohol Abuse and Alcoholism (NIAAA) reports "...approximately one-half of all sexual assault victims report that they were drinking alcohol at the time of the assault."[52]

- In one American Medical Association survey, 26 percent of U. S. parents felt it was okay for teens to drink alcohol at home.[53]

- "In 2005, 23 percent of the young drivers (15 to 20 years old) involved in fatal crashes had a [blood alcohol level exceeding the "safe" limit]."[54]

- "Nearly one in four teens ... say their own parents have supplied them with alcohol ..."[55]

Did You Know?

Alcohol is a Drug!
If not treated as such, its effects can lead to:

1. Cancer caused by permanent damage to vital organs
2. Gastrointestinal illness, irritation or ulcers
3. Chronic Candida or yeast overgrowth
4. Sexual dysfunction
5. An overworked immune system
6. Liver disease
7. Malnutrition
8. Depression and anxiety

The liver processes 95% of the alcohol you consume. Alcohol converts to fat in the body and excess alcohol intake eventually overwhelms the liver with fatty deposits. Continued alcohol abuse can thus lead to a dysfunctional liver.

Alcohol is also associated with many gastrointestinal disorders. Alcohol damages the mucosal lining and disrupts the enzyme function of the upper gastrointestinal tract. Also, more hydrochloric acid is created by the stomach, leading to inflammation and possible stomach ulcers. Also, with regular alcohol consumption, foods are not alkalized properly, and this can result in leaky gut syndrome. Alcohol also impairs the body's ability to absorb many essential nutrients such as Vitamins A, B, D, E, and K as well as the minerals calcium, zinc, and folic acid.

DOCTOR'S NOTE:
Hangovers are actually caused by dehydration from alcohol consumption coupled with toxic effects from the fermentation within your digestive system. Some drinkers claim taking oxygen-based colon cleansers after drinking can reduce the noticeable effects of hangovers.

How to Eliminate Toxins from Alcohol

- Eliminate or drastically reduce all alcohol consumption.

- Detoxify and cleanse your body. Once your body is cleansed, the cravings for alcohol should disappear.

- Reduce drinking habits to a maximum of one night weekly. The safest alcoholic beverages are unfiltered beer or vodka.

- Try drinking extra water with raw organic Apple Cider Vinegar instead of an alcoholic beverage.

- If alcohol abuse is a problem, seek professional help.

- Supplement with the calcium orotate and zinc orotate.

- Cleansing your colon weekly can reduce the effects alcohol has on the intestinal mucosa, preventing leaky gut syndrome and alcohol induced fermentation of foods.

- Remember how alcohol makes you feel the next morning.

- Educate your children on the short and long-term effects of alcohol consumption. Do them a favor and do not let them drink. Alcohol is a drug and poison!

- To detoxify the liver of fatty deposits, I recommend three consecutive liver/gallbladder cleansing sessions. See *Chapter 12—Dr. Group's Liver/Gallbladder Cleanse.*

- Regular exercise increases your endorphins, giving you a "natural high".

- Take a high quality oxygen based intestinal cleanser before bed, especially after alcohol consumption.

Closing Thought

You might be thinking, "It's so difficult to follow all these rules about eating and drinking. It's not my fault fast food and junk food is all that's out there!"

Do you remember Charles de Coti-Marsh who wrote about the benefits of eating raw, organic foods? Perhaps you can take some inspiration from his advice, *"If beneficial results can be obtained by altering our diets from bad foods to good foods, at a time when the civilised world suffers such painful and formerly incurable diseases, then let every citizen attack by letters to the Press, and by refusal to purchase harmful, so-called eatables offered as foods. Raise the standard of foods, especially for children, and watch the standard of health and energy just grow in them week by week."*[56]

In other words, it's time to become proactive about your health and demand real change!

CHAPTER 7

CHAPTER EIGHT

HOW TO REDUCE INTESTINAL TOXINS FROM AIR AND WATER

Oxygen is the single most abundant element in our bodies next to water. We can live for several weeks without food and for several days without water, but the human brain dies after just a few minutes without oxygen.

Nearly half of the world's oxygen supply comes from trees, grasses, and other plants. The other half comes from phytoplankton in the oceans. Unfortunately, both of these sources are being depleted by humanity's destructive habits. The burning of coal and fossil fuels

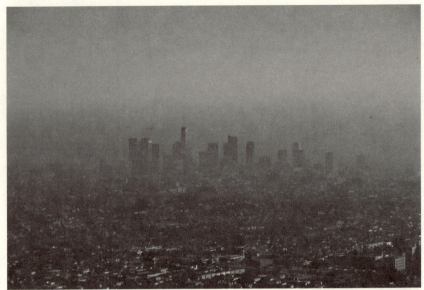

Fig. IV: Smog trapped over Los Angeles

releases carbon dioxide into the atmosphere, thinning the protective ozone layer. An excess of ultraviolet B radiation is allowed through areas of the ozone layer that have become too thin. The ultraviolet B rays infiltrate the ocean and disrupt the phytoplankton's ability to produce oxygen. Moreover, some estimates state at least 100 acres of trees are cut down every minute. The loss of forestry further depletes oxygen levels and allows carbon dioxide levels to rise.

Exposure to an excess of carbon dioxide prevents red blood cells in the lungs from extracting oxygen to deliver it to vital organs. Oxygen is required to oxidize chemicals and other toxins within the body, which makes it an indispensable part of maintaining a healthy, functional colon. Environmental health researcher Sara Shannon theorizes, "… we may have originally evolved in an atmosphere of 38 percent oxygen. But now, due to the loss of forests and ocean plankton, our two sources of oxygen production, measurements of oxygen as low as 12 percent and 15 percent have been made in heavily industrialized areas. This oxygen-depleted condition is a contributing cause of the generalized lack of well-being that many are experiencing. And it does not look good for the future. We need oxygen to live!"[57]

How Can Air Cause a Toxic Colon?

The average person takes in about 30,000 breaths each day. Unfortunately, every one of them is potentially harmful due to the poor quality of our environment. The air we breathe isn't just losing its vital oxygen content—it's also filled with harmful toxins! Remember—the body depends on receiving enough oxygen to carry out toxin removal. How can the colon possibly eliminate chemicals and other poisonous material when the body is simultaneously hindered with too many toxins and not enough oxygen?

By this point, you are somewhat familiar with many of the common toxins we encounter in our lives. The harmful effects of carbon dioxide, sulphur dioxide, and countless other chemicals created by modern industries (mining, quarrying, transportation, power generation, agriculture, etc.) are well documented. We know these chemicals are bad, but a single person has very little ability to stop the spread of pollutants. Instead of focusing on the obvious outdoor pollutants made by an industrialized world, this chapter will highlight an array of some of the less obvious toxins permeating the air of our indoor environments e.g. our homes, schools, and office buildings.

The scariest part is–most of the toxins we absorb from the air are found indoors. Think about how much time most of us spend indoors at home, work, school, while shopping, etc. These places are often virtual stews of smoke, pet dander, paint fumes, mold, mildew, and billions of microorganisms.

Important Facts about Indoor Air Quality

- The average American spends about 90% of their life indoors.

- "Every year, indoor air pollution is responsible for the death of 1.6 million people - that's one death every 20 seconds…due to pneumonia, chronic respiratory disease and lung cancer…"[58]

Important Facts about Indoor Air Quality

- Though the word "pollution" often conjures images of smog and litter everywhere, indoor air is up to 10 times more contaminated than outdoor air.

- Most American buildings are designed to be airtight to save money on heating and cooling, but this hyper-sealing allows pollutants to stay trapped inside and also prevents the admission of natural purifying agents such as negative ions and ozone from outside air.

- Heavily insulated homes harbor more allergens than homes with less insulation.

- Playing and crawling on a typical floor exposes babies to contaminants such as mold, mildew, and dust mites. Just one day of exposure introduces the equivalent of four cigarettes into an infant's lungs.[59]

- Indoor air quality is one of the leading environmental health concerns in the United States.[60]

The amount of colon toxins derived from indoor air is really quite alarming, especially considering how much time most of us spend indoors. These toxins can be chemically based or generated by living organisms (e.g. animal dander or mold spores). Where these toxins come from is important so you know how to eliminate these nasty contaminants lurking in your household.

You may be wondering how these airborne toxins enter your colon. Your airways are lined with mucous and when you breathe, toxins can adhere to the mucus linings in sinuses and bronchial passages. This mucous (along with the toxins) then drains into the throat where it is inadvertently swallowed, thus transferring toxins into the stomach and eventually into the entire intestinal tract and colon.

DOCTOR'S NOTE:
Not all toxins will wind up in mucous—some of them will be absorbed through the lungs and go directly into the bloodstream.

How Do Chemical Toxins Present an Indoor Air Hazard?

It may be difficult to believe that indoor air is more hazardous than outdoor air. How can that be, you say, when refineries, large trucks, and passenger autos emit dangerous pollutants all the time? In outdoor environments, toxic chemicals dissipate through the air. However, think about the design of most indoor environments (such as office buildings)—four walls, a floor, a ceiling, and maybe a few windows that don't even open. Airborne chemicals are literally trapped inside homes and other modern structures with nowhere to go but into you and your family's bodies.

What kinds of chemical toxins permeate indoor air?

According to the EPA, "By volume, paint is the largest category of waste brought into household hazardous waste collection programs."[61] Paint, especially older paints, can be extremely hazardous to the human body. If you have any old paint cans sitting around in the garage, it's a good idea to take them to an authorized collection center.

Lead-based paints were commonly used until 1977 when the U.S. Consumer Product Safety Commission finally banned them, but only after many people (including babies) had ingested the toxic substance from exposure to paint chips or dust. Mercury, also very toxic, was regularly added to preserve many latex paints until 1990, when the EPA banned its use in indoor paints.[62] A single breath of mercury fumes can poison the body and trigger a wide range of symptoms such as abdominal pain and diarrhea.

Now that lead and mercury have been banned from their ingredients, indoor paints are completely safe again, right? Well, not exactly. Most paints (even latex paints) release chemicals known as Volatile Organic

Compounds (VOC's) and these can be extremely toxic once airborne. VOC's have high vapor pressures and this allows them to quickly evaporate within the atmosphere.

Millions of people are inhaling these toxic compounds on a daily basis. As VOC's build up in the body, they can lead to eye, nose, and throat irritation, headaches, loss of coordination, nausea, damage to the liver, kidneys, and central nervous system. **Some VOC's have even been shown to cause cancer in animals.**

VOC levels are generally estimated to be ten times greater in indoor environments than in outdoor spaces. Freshly applied indoor paint can actually produce up to a thousand times more VOC's! However, paint isn't the only source of these toxins. Tons of common products emit these harmful gases. The EPA provides us with examples of commonly used items: "…mineral spirits, toluene or xylene … enamels, varnishes, shellacs, lacquers, stains, and sealers … latex and water colors."[63]

Eliminating exposure to all products containing VOC's is probably impossible, but you can certainly take steps to limit that exposure in your household. Remember, the more toxins you can eliminate the better your health will become.

How to Eliminate Toxins from VOC's (Volatile Organic Compounds)

- Purchase non-toxic, VOC-free paints from alternative companies instead of those manufactured by large corporations. (See www.greenplanetpaints.com)
- Switch to non-toxic household products. Open windows or run exhaust fans to reduce the circulation of fumes within your home.

- Remove old or unneeded chemical products from your home. Dispose of them at a designated drop-off for toxic household wastes.

- Read product labels in their entirety for ingredients and instructions. Be on the lookout for the VOC "methylene chloride", especially in paint stripper and spray-paint.

- Use a quality air purification system that incorporates UV, negative ions, and HEPA filter technology. Surround Air™ and Way Healthier Home™ are both excellent brands.

- Avoid dry-cleaning your clothes or find a cleaner that uses natural agents instead of chemicals which produce VOC vapors.

- Always use a mask and gloves when handling any VOC-containing products.

- Cleanse your intestines, liver, and gallbladder regularly to help prevent long-term damage to your body and internal organs. See Chapter 12.

- For more information, see "Paint" and "Air Purification" in the *Resources* section.

How Does Tobacco Smoke Damage the Colon?

There's not much of a debate anymore about the toxic effects of tobacco smoke on the lungs. It's common knowledge that the additives and chemicals in cigarette smoke cause lung cancer. However, not as widely reported is the link between tobacco usage and colorectal cancer. Tobacco smoke delivers carcinogens to the colon and increases the size of polyps. The larger a polyp becomes, the greater the risk of it metastasizing into cancer. In fact, smoking "…may increase the risk of death from

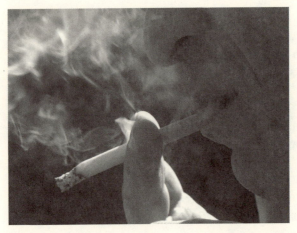

cancer of the colon or rectum by up to 43%."[64]

This seems like an easy fix, right? Avoid colon toxins from tobacco smoke by Not Smoking. Sounds reasonable, but unfortunately, the factor of secondhand smoke must also be considered. Exposure to secondhand smoke, also known as environmental tobacco smoke (ETS), can cause toxic buildup in people who don't smoke. Secondhand smoke can even lead to colon cancer by damaging genes of anyone exposed to it.

The risk of getting cancer from secondhand smoke is approximately 100 times greater than the risk from outdoor contaminants alone. This is especially unsettling in a society where nearly one in four people smoke![65] The nonsmoker can be exposed to tobacco smoke in the workplace, at home, in restaurants and bars, and in other public places. However, I'm glad to say, many metropolitan governments are now enacting measures to ban cigarette smoke in all interior environments.

So far, fourteen states have implemented significant anti-smoking laws. Nine of these states ban smoking in nearly all workplaces. This is encouraging but we still have a long way to go. Children and non-smoking adults continue to suffer from the ill effects of secondhand smoke in their own homes due to the presence of others whom smoke. Around 60% of children under the age of five live in or visit a home with at least one smoker. Children are especially sensitive to secondhand smoke, as their developing organs are more easily damaged. Protect yourself and your family from the dangers of environmental tobacco smoke!

How to Eliminate Toxins from Tobacco Smoke

- Quit smoking! You may need a support group to help you.

- Avoid smoking inside the home. Go outside to smoke (at least 100 feet away from the house).

- When you have the urge to smoke, distract yourself with an activity of some kind or take a short walk.

- Ask visitors to step out of the home if they must smoke.

- When going to restaurants and other public places, ask ahead of time if they are smoke-free or have designated non-smoking areas.

- Never smoke near a child, not even outdoors.

- If quitting smoking altogether is impossible, smoke all-natural or organic tobacco.

- Detoxify your body with an intestinal, liver, gallbladder, and heavy metal cleanse program.

- Repeat the following affirmation throughout the day: "I am proud to be a non-smoker".

Toxins from Biological Contaminants in the Air

The EPA defines biological contaminants as "living organisms or their derivatives," and these include mold, mildew, bacteria, dust mites, animal dander, and viruses. Regular exposure to any of these contaminants can cause toxic buildup in the colon, which can lead to the onset of serious diseases. Children, the elderly, and people with weakened immune systems are especially susceptible to airborne biological contaminants.

Many people commonly suffer from outdoor allergens like pollen, cedar, and ragweed. At least as many people are allergic to a range of toxic biological contaminants found indoors as well. Let's take a look at some of the most common indoor organisms and learn how to eliminate them from your environment.

Do You Have Mold and Mildew in Your Home?

Think about the last time you cleaned your bathroom. You probably used a toxic bathroom cleaner to scrub some of that nasty black mold and mildew off the tiles in the shower. Guess what—your body was bombarded with the chemicals from the cleaner on top of the airborne mold spores freed from the various surfaces of the shower stall.

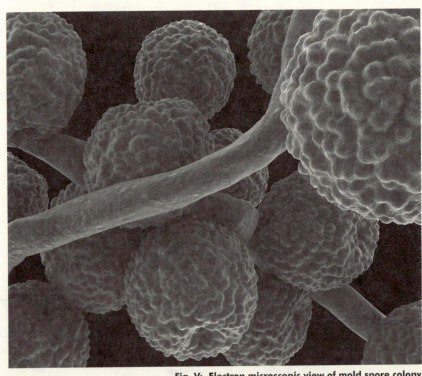

Fig. V: Electron microscopic view of mold spore colony

What is the difference between mold and mildew? They're practically the same thing and the terms are often used interchangeably. Mold is microscopic fungi that proliferate in damp areas. Mold growing in a shower or bathtub is usually referred to as mildew. Mildew and mold reproduce via airborne spores that are constantly seeking more moisture. This is why mold is found in sections of a home that are likely to have damp surfaces such as walls (inside and out), cabinets, and any other poorly vented areas that can trap condensation and provide a breeding ground for mold.

DOCTOR'S NOTE:
Mold and their spores may account for almost all chronic sinus infections.

Mold occurs naturally outdoors, so it's expected that some airborne mold spores will invariably make their way into indoor environments. This is normal, but the problem stems from the indoor mold colonies that multiply.

Envirochex, an indoor-environment consultant firm, explains, "When these organisms are allowed to grow in a closed indoor environment, they can release millions of spores causing indoor levels to reach concentrations that are hundreds of times higher than outdoors ... levels that can be detrimental to even healthy people."[66] Mold toxin exposure has been linked to respiratory ailments, as well as nausea and diarrhea. To greatly reduce mold and mildew exposure, follow the recommendations below.

How to Eliminate Toxins from Mold and Mildew

- Controlling moisture is the key to regulating indoor mold!
- Wipe away leaks, spills, or condensation as soon as you notice them. Removing the moisture quickly will decrease the likelihood of mold reproduction.

How to Eliminate Toxins from Mold and Mildew (contd.)

- Use a dehumidifier to help clear moisture out of the air. If you live in a high humidity area, dehumidify the house at least twice a week.

- Run your air conditioner as needed but change or clean the filter often.

- Ventilate the bathroom with a fan while showering.

- In Australia, Tea Tree Oil is commonly used in ventilation systems to control bacteria and mold growth.

- Have your home tested for mold spores, particularly if you live in a humid area. (See www.homemoldtestkit.com)

- Use a high quality air purification system that includes UV, negative ions, and HEPA filter technology. The Germicidal UV lamp is the most effective air purification method available for destroying microorganisms like viruses, bacteria, and fungi (including mold).

- For more information, see "Air Purification" and "Mold and Mildew Control" in the *Resources* section.

Colon Toxins from Pet Dander

Pet or animal dander is similar to dandruff from humans. Dander is just dead skin cells that have come loose. Older pets tend to shed more dander than younger ones because their skin is drier. Dander can accumulate all over the house but is usually concentrated in areas where the animal sleeps such as carpet, beds, sofas, and other upholstered furniture. When these skin cells become airborne, they can be inhaled or swallowed. Remember—virtually all the toxins you are exposed to on a daily basis enter your bloodstream through the intestinal lining.

It's estimated the pet population exceeds 100 million in America alone. Furthermore, up to 30 percent of people with allergies are specifically allergic to furred or feathered animals ... but many of these people actually own pets![67] That's an awful lot of people needlessly breathing in toxic particles every day. If someone is severely allergic to pet dander, it's best to keep their home environment (and especially pet areas) as clean as possible.

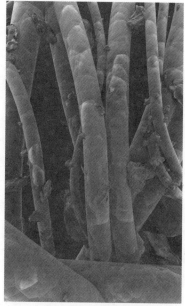

Fig. VI: Pet dander in carpet

Animal lovers, don't despair! By following the recommendations in the chart below, you can greatly reduce the amount of pet dander that you might inhale.

How to Eliminate Indoor Toxins from Pet Dander

- If possible, keep your pets outside or in a designated room of your home. Place an air purifier in that room.
- Designate at least one room, such as the bedroom, to be completely pet-free.

How to Eliminate Indoor Toxins from Pet Dander (contd.)

- Wash your hands thoroughly after petting any animal.

- Bathe your pet weekly with a high quality, chemical-free pet shampoo, preferably outdoors. This practice alone can reduce pet dander by up to 80 percent.

- Brush your pet outside 3 or more times weekly to reduce loose dander.

- Keep pets off the furniture and carpeted areas as much as possible.

- Change or clean the filter of your air conditioner monthly to prevent dander recirculation.

- Vacuum and wash all bedding frequently using an all-natural laundry detergent and a vacuum with a HEPA filter.

- Use an excellent air purification system that includes UV, negative ion, and HEPA filtration. Surround Air™ and Way Healthier Home™ are both excellent brands.

- Cleanse your colon regularly to help purge accumulated allergens from your bowels.

- For more information, see "Air Purification" and "Pet Dander", in the *Resources* section.

Colon Toxins from Dust Mites

Did You Know?

Your mattress can host anywhere from 100,000 to 10 million of these parasitic creatures! They can also account for 10% of the total weight of pillows used over six years. These numbers are even more disturbing when you consider that roughly one-third of your life is spent in bed.

Only a fraction of a millimeter long, the almost invisible mite permeates dust in homes all over the world. Closely related to ticks and spiders, these eight-legged creatures live and breed in bedding, curtains, rugs, carpeting, stuffed animals, couches, and old clothing. Dust mites feed on

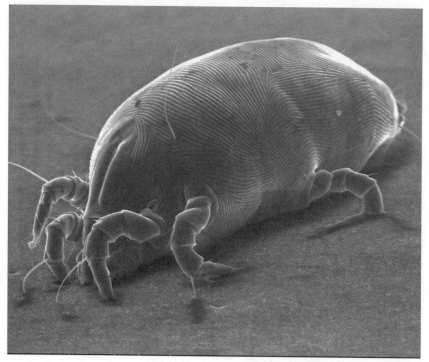

Fig. VII: Magnified view of a dust mite

animal dander and dead skin scales from humans. The life span of a dust mite is two to four months. In that time, a single mite can produce about 2,000 protein-containing droppings—the actual cause of "dust allergies". These droppings are highly toxic and, when inhaled or swallowed, they can accumulate in your sinuses and intestinal tract and cause immune system overload.

Can you believe just one ounce of house dust can support 30,000 dust mites! A study published in the *Journal of Allergy and Clinical Immunology* found that most American homes (just over 84 percent) contain detectable amounts of dust mites in bedding.[68] It was also discovered that older homes, homes with mold, and homes with high humidity in the bedrooms usually have the highest levels of dust mites.

Research at Clemson University suggests dust mites are the leading cause of perennial allergic rhinitis.[69] Dust mites are impossible to view without a microscope. However, you can decrease your exposure to these toxic organisms with a few simple practices.

How to Eliminate Toxins from Dust Mites

- Use a dehumidifier 2 to 3 times weekly in your home to reduce moisture. Dust mites are attracted to warm, humid areas, so it is a good idea to keep the humidity under 50 percent.

- Check your bedding for dust mites in 10 minutes using the Mite-T-Fast™ home test kit.

- Use wood blinds and shades instead of cloth drapes or curtains.

- Buy new hypoallergenic pillows every year to prevent the accumulation of droppings, or use dust-mite free organic cotton mattress and pillow casings.

- Wash all bedding weekly in very hot water (130 degrees Fahrenheit) with a natural laundry detergent. Add essential oils, tea tree, or eucalyptus to the spin cycle when washing bedding, curtains, rugs, etc. This will help kill any lingering dust mites. Dry bedding on a high heat cycle.

- Replace carpet with non-toxic hardwood flooring or non-toxic wool carpeting. If this is not a feasible option, use all natural carpet cleaning supplies to kill residual mites.

- Vacuum often but make sure people with severe dust allergies leave the house while doing so. Use a vacuum with a HEPA filter and change the filter often.

- Use a quality air purification system with UV, negative ion, and HEPA filter technology.

- Cleanse your digestive tract regularly to help make sure your body is free of parasites.

For more information, see "Dust Mites", "Bedding" and "Pillows," in the *Resources* section.

Are You Suffering From Sick Building Syndrome?

Have you ever become nauseous, achy, or dizzy after spending an extended amount of time in a specific building? It's possible you experienced Sick Building Syndrome (SBS) or Building Related Illness (BRI). Although both of these two conditions are generally associated with the workplace, an important distinction should be made. Sick Building Syndrome occurs when inhabitants of a particular building report health symptoms seemingly linked to actual time spent in that building. However, no specific illness can be pinpointed. Building Related Illness, on the other hand, characterizes an occupant's diagnosable condition

Sick Building/House

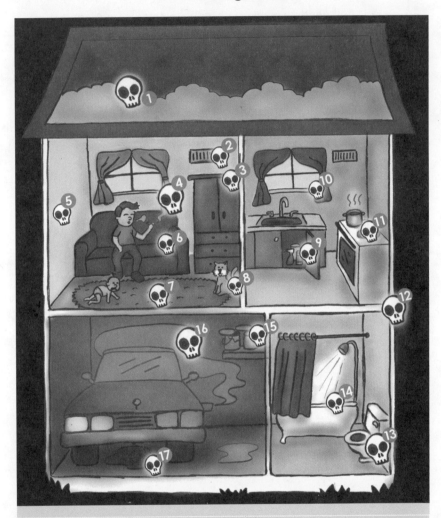

A Variety Of Common Toxins Found in Homes

1. Synthetic Insulation
2. Poor Air Circulation
3. Lack of Fresh Air
4. Smoke
5. Paint Fumes
6. Dustmites
7. Synthetic Carpet Outgassing
8. Pet Dander
9. Toxic Household Cleaners
10. Fabric Outgassing
11. Natural Gas/CO2
12. Construction Materials
13. Bacteria from Toilet Bowl
14. Mold/Mildew
15. Lead or Toxic Paint
16. Carbon Monoxide
17. Oil & Gas Fumes

that can be directly connected to the toxic agents pervading the air of the building.

Building occupants complaining of temporary symptoms such as fatigue, dizziness, nausea, headache, dry cough, concentration difficulties, or eye, nose, and throat irritation are probably suffering from Sick Building Syndrome. In this situation, most symptoms subside after leaving the particular building. Occupants suffering prolonged symptoms even after leaving a building are more likely to have Building Related Illness. Symptoms of BRI include chest tightness, cough, chills, fever, and muscle aches. Poor indoor air quality is a major contributor of both conditions. Insufficient ventilation systems, toxic VOCs, and biological contaminants all contribute to a less than desirable environment. It's estimated 1 in 3 buildings are hazardous enough to human health to be labeled as "sick."[70]

Let's Review!

Daily airborne contaminants like mold, mildew, smoke, VOCs, dust mites, and pet dander all contribute to the number of toxins entering your body every day! Luckily, you can improve the air quality of indoor environments. Follow the suggestions below and start protecting yourself and family. Eliminating airborne pollutants significantly reduces your daily exposure to toxins.

Extra Tips for Cleansing Toxins from the Air

- Place live toxin-absorbing plants in each room of your home and office. Boston ferns, Peace lilies, Arrowhead vines, Goldon Pothos, English Ivy, Spider plants, Dracaenas, Areca palms, and Chrysanthemums are excellent choices.

- Use natural instead of chemically based air fresheners. You can dilute the following essential oils in distilled water to spray

> ### Extra Tips for Cleansing Toxins from the Air (contd.)
>
> around the home or office: Tea tree, Citronella, Lavender, Orange, and Lemongrass.
>
> - Opening windows during a rainstorm will provide circulation of fresh, clean oxygen-rich air.

How To Eliminate Intestinal Toxins from Water

Water promotes efficient bowel function by decreasing the risk of constipation and maintaining regular waste elimination. Water is also necessary for flushing toxins from the liver, kidneys, and colon. Equally critical is water's benefit for nutrient absorption, particularly when taking water-soluble vitamins. When the body's water supply is insufficient, the colon attempts to make up for it by absorbing water from feces. Fecal matter without water—what does that become? Constipation! Stools will be harder to eliminate and may irritate and damage the intestinal lining. A chronically dehydrated colon will not produce healthy bowel movements and can lead to life-threatening bowel conditions.

Water is the secret to life! Every living thing, even rocks, depends on water to survive. The human body is composed of about 75 percent water and 30 percent solid matter. Both blood and the brain are approximately 80 percent water. Our lungs, which are so closely associated with air, are actually 90 percent water! Therefore, it's no surprise that we begin to feel ill whenever our bodies are deprived of even a little water.

Nearly all of the body's internal processes (including digestion and waste elimination) require water. Did you know the amount of water we drink (or don't drink) each day plays a major role in whether or not we develop a toxic colon?

Why is Water So Important?

Many people consume plenty of liquids throughout the day, but not enough clean, refreshing water! A significant difference exists between drinking sodas and drinking water, especially when it comes to your digestive health. Our bodies are not made of sodas, coffee, or alcohol—they're made of pure water! Drinking these beverages throughout the day dehydrates the body and increases the amount of stress placed

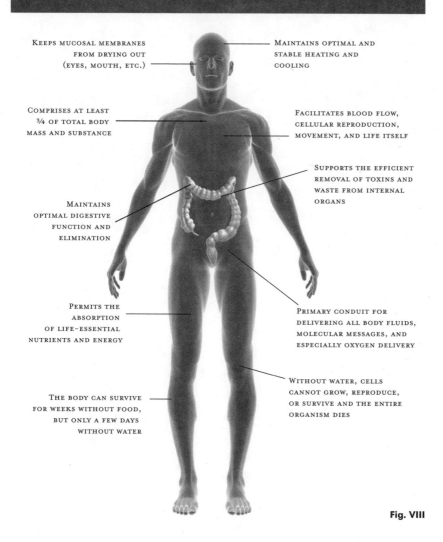

Fig. VIII

on internal cleansing organs like the colon, liver and kidneys. To put it another way, anything you drink besides water requires water to break it down. Despite this simple logic, *a large portion of the population continues to drink unhealthful beverages instead of water and they are chronically dehydrated!*

Sadly, even people who drink enough water are often obtaining it from contaminated sources (such as public utilities), the kitchen faucet and deceptively labeled bottled water. The EPA lists over eighty "regulated" contaminants found in tap water such as chlorine, fluoride, arsenic, and numerous pesticides. This figure doesn't even include unregulated toxins such as perchlorate (a chemical found in rocket fuel!).

You might be saying, "I drink bottled water, so I don't need to read this section."

- What about the toxic water the cows, pigs, fish, or chickens drink that ends up in the meat you eventually eat?
- What about the water used to grow the vegetables and fruit you enjoy each day?
- What about the water you use to wash your dishes, clothes, towels, and bedding?
- What about the water you swim in or bathe in?

All of these sources and more can expose you to toxic chemicals in water!

Drinking tap water overwhelms the intestines with toxins and prevents essential nutrients from being absorbed into the body. Even if you avoid tap water, you're still not exempt from exposure to toxins. Simply taking a shower can expose your body to toxic chemicals. As a matter of fact, while showering for just fifteen minutes, your body can absorb the same amount of toxins as drinking seven glasses of tap water! Moreover, the heat from a steaming shower causes your skin pores to dilate and absorb even more of those toxins directly. Likewise, if you're lounging next to a pool on a hot day, your pores will dilate. You will notice this because you'll begin sweating. Then, when you jump into the pool, your skin is going to absorb high levels of chlorine through those wide-open pores.

Unfortunately, we're not protecting ourselves by drinking bottled water either. It's well documented that several popular water manufacturers have actually been bottling plain old tap water and selling it to the public all along. You can't always trust labels stating "drinking water" or "spring water"—they may not be free of harmful chemicals. Just because a clever marketing campaign makes use of images of pristine mountain streams and waterfalls, don't believe for an instant the water actually originated there! As always, read the label and research the manufacturing facility and its standards.

How do all of these chemicals and other toxins in water affect the colon, and consequently, the overall health of the body? Let's review the harmful effects of common toxins found in our water supply—arsenic, fluoride, chlorine, and others.

Most water contains Arsenic!

Arsenic is an extremely toxic heavy metal that damages the human nervous system, causes birth defects, and leads to several types of cancer. This substance is poisonous if inhaled but the primary mode of contamination worldwide is through the water supply. The International Agency for Research on Cancer (IARC) has labeled arsenic as a Category 1 carcinogen, which basically means the chemical is definitely (as opposed to possibly) a cancer-causing agent. Fact—arsenic is number one on the 2005 CERCLA Harmful Substance List according to the Agency for Toxic Substances & Disease Registry (ATSDR).[71]

Much research has confirmed a link between long-term consumption of arsenic-polluted water and the risk of developing multiple cancers, including colon cancer, and lowered mental development in children. However, symptoms may not appear for years later as it takes time for this toxic metal to accumulate in the body.[72] The National Resources Defense Council (NRDC) estimates "…as many as 56 million people in the 25 states reviewed by the U. S. Environmental Protection Agency … have been drinking water with unsafe levels of arsenic..."![73] Arsenic enters the body through the intestinal tract and, if not eliminated, can contribute to a weakened immune system and bowel disease.

Levels of arsenic in the environment can increase with natural events such as volcanic activity, rock erosion, and forest fires; but human actions can also release arsenic, often in extremely hazardous amounts. Every year, industrial pollution accounts for the release of thousands of pounds of the deadly chemical. Wood preservatives account for 90 percent of the arsenic used in American industry, but it can also be found in paints, metals, prescription and recreational drugs, soaps, and fertilizers, and occurs as a byproduct of mining, copper smelting, and coal burning.

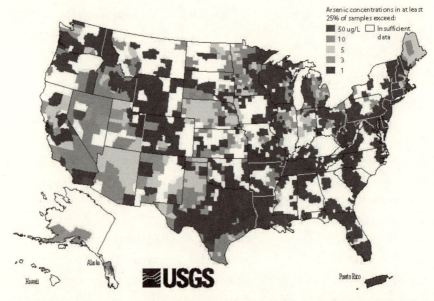

Fig. IX: 2001 United States Geological Survey – Arsenic concentration in U.S. homes.

Ground water sources can contain especially high concentrations of arsenic since the metal can leech out of adjacent rocks. The EPA has set a standard of 10 μg/L (ten micrograms per liter) as an acceptable level for tap water.[74] This means it's not safe to drink water with arsenic concentrations higher than 10 parts per billion. Water systems in the Midwest, New England, and some western states (Oregon and Nevada) often exceed this standard.

>
> *Did You Know?*
>
> The EPA has reported that "... roughly five percent, or 3,000 community water systems serving 11 million people, will have to take corrective action to lower the current levels of arsenic in their drinking water." [75]

We know arsenic contributes to cancer and other colon diseases, but let's learn about other toxins found in water. After that, I will give you several powerful tips on preventing and eliminating these toxins from your water sources.

Most water contains Fluoride!

Fluoride is one of the most toxic substances known to man; yet based on its inclusion in virtually every brand of toothpaste, the American Dental Association believes it's okay to use fluoride for preventative dental care. Other products, such as bottled water, infant formulas, and even vitamin supplements, now contain fluoride! In 2002, nearly 90 percent of the U.S. population was supplied water via public water systems, and around 67 percent of that number received fluoridated water. This occurred in spite of the fact, "No statistically significant differences were found in the decay rates of permanent teeth or the percentages of decay-free children in the fluoridated, non-fluoridated, and partially fluoridated areas."[76]

Material Safety Data Sheets (MSDS) typically label sodium fluoride as "... toxic by ingestion, inhalation and skin contact" and that PPE (personal protection equipment) for handling should include safety glasses and gloves.[77] **Fluorides are more toxic than lead and only slightly less poisonous than arsenic ... and these toxins can enter your body from brushing your teeth or rinsing with many popular dental care products!** Fluoride compounds are still purposefully added to water in many areas (in a process known as fluoridation) and is used in most brands of toothpaste to help prevent tooth decay. However, fluoride has never been proven to significantly aid in protecting teeth from the

COUNTERTHINK

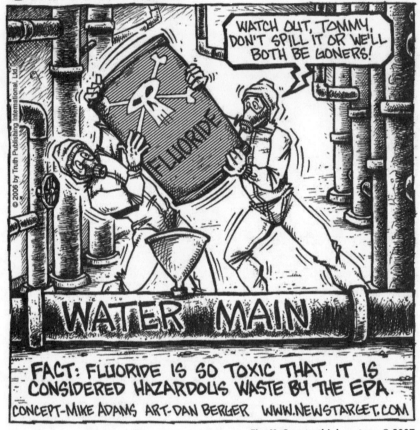

Fig. X: Counterthink cartoon © 2007

development of cavities.

Every year Poison Control centers receive thousands of calls from people reporting excessive consumption of fluoride-containing products (vitamins, toothpaste, mouthwash, etc.). Fluoride poisoning severely damages the body and can be fatal. This lethal chemical creates a toxic state that can cause a variety of harmful effects.

Potential Results of Consuming Fluoridated Water

- Bone and uterine cancer
- Lowered IQ (especially in young children)

- Birth defects
- Perinatal death
- Immune system suppression
- Osteoarthritis
- Skeletal Fluorosis (leading to brittle teeth and bones)
- Gastrointestinal disorders
- Essential enzyme inhibition
- Acute poisoning

The practice of water fluoridation has been rejected or banned in several countries including: China, Austria, Belgium, Finland, Germany, Denmark, Norway, Sweden, the Netherlands, Hungary, and Japan. Nearly all of Europe's water supply is fluoride-free, and thankfully, many American communities are realizing this is the healthier choice. More than 45 U.S. cities have rejected the process of water fluoridation since 1990. Now, if the remaining 30,000 will follow along, the entire nation will have access to fluoride-free water.

Did You Know?

Five percent of the world's population still receives fluoridated water and over half of those people reside in North America!

With all this knowledge and current research demonstrating the harmful effects of fluoride, can you believe a company (DS Waters of America Inc.) would actually market bottled water for children containing this toxin? Nursery®, for infants, actually advertises on the label that it has "added fluoride"![78] Furthermore, this company goes on to state, **"If you make the choice not to breastfeed, you can still give your baby all the nutrients he/she needs with commercial formula."**[79]

Of course, the manufacturer would stand to profit from this advice as they subtly suggest "Nursery®" can be ideal for mixing with baby formulas. To support their position, the company misconstrues "recommendations" from the American Academy of Pediatrics and the FDA that chemically synthesized formula is just as good as real breastmilk. In fact, DS Waters' "research" was obviously obtained from the website of a doctor whose tradition-oriented childcare theories have been all but invalidated, misguided, and just plain harmful to your child's development![80]

Our poor children are being poisoned and they don't even know it! It really bothers me that so many parents do not even bother researching what they feed to their kids. Twenty years from now, when all of these substances have been banned as cancer-causing agents, many young adults will be asking, "Mom, Dad, Why did you feed me all of these toxic chemicals?" What will you say to your child? "Sorry, the manufacturer said it was OK"?

With that being said, the great news is—the human body can detoxify and repair itself at a rapid rate. So it's not too late to cleanse your body and begin avoiding these toxic chemicals!

Most water contains Chlorine!

Yet another chemical contaminating nationwide water supplies is chlorine. Chlorine is a disinfectant used to kill waterborne diseases such as cholera, dysentery, E. coli and typhoid and has been used regularly in municipal water treatment facilities for more than a century. **It's estimated over 200 million Americans have at least marginally chlorinated water pumped into their homes every day for washing clothes, bathing, cooking, and drinking.**

Chlorine may be effective at eliminating many pathogens, but its presence in drinking water does more harm than good. When chlorine is added to water, it bonds with other natural compounds to form Trihalomethanes (THM's). These chlorine byproducts trigger the production of free radicals in the body, thereby causing extensive cell damage.

According to a study published in the *Journal of the National Cancer Institute,* Chlorine or chloramine was administered daily in the drinking water of rats, and the rats subsequently developed tumors in their liver, kidney, and intestines. The study determined "...organic byproducts of chlorination are the chemicals of greatest concern for the carcinogenic potential of chlorinated drinking water."[81] **If animals are developing chlorine-related cancerous growths, then why is the government continuing to provide chlorinated water to its citizens?**

Chlorinated water can enter our bodies in more than just the obvious ways. We can inhale chlorine in gas form, as steam from a hot shower, and/or absorb it through our skin! Taking a hot shower is a routine way to contaminate your body. Heat causes pores in the skin to expand. This factor, coupled with chlorine's ability to vaporize quickly, allows the toxin to be absorbed into the body very quickly. The chlorine vapors are also inhaled at the same time, thus burdening the body with even greater amounts. This doesn't affect just the individual taking the shower. Chlorine vapors from the bathroom can spread throughout the home and expose others to its toxic effects! Inhaling chlorine is a serious health risk since it can be absorbed directly into the bloodstream without being filtered by the kidneys.

Did You Know?

Chlorine gas was used as a form of chemical warfare in World War I. That's how toxic this stuff really is!

In a study appearing in *Environmental Health Perspectives,* M. Kanarek and T. Young found that the consumption of chlorinated water significantly correlates to the onset of brain and colon cancer. Kanarek and Young also observed a higher risk for bladder and gastrointestinal cancer.[82]

An even more alarming study published in the *American Journal of Public Health* estimates a 95% risk of developing cancer from regular consumption of chlorinated tap water![83]

It's simply ridiculous to continue chlorinating water for consumer use. This toxic substance penetrates the body's critical systems whether you are taking a bath, relaxing in a hot tub, drinking a glass of water, or having fun in a backyard pool.

Did You Know?

In the 1984 Summer Olympics, European swim teams refused to compete until chlorination procedures were halted. Instead, the Olympic pool was ozonated to prevent the growth of bacteria.

Many nations understand chlorine is detrimental to the health of its citizens and that safe alternatives exist for disinfecting water. The use of ozone (O_3) in water treatment facilities has proven to be an effective practice for killing harmful organisms. Even some municipalities in the United States have replaced chlorination with ozonation, but the improvement is not nearly as widespread as it should be.

DOCTOR'S NOTE:

I personally use the ECOsmarte® system in my pool, which uses copper ions and ozone to purify the water. Plus, I receive the added benefit of swimming in oxygen-rich water. Oxygen naturally detoxifies the body and is also absorbed into the bloodstream for use by the body.

You can learn more about the ECOsmarte® system at: www.ecosmarte.com

Most water contains other Toxic Contaminants as well!

Perchlorate is a toxic compound manufactured primarily as an oxidizer in rocket fuel although it can also be found in fireworks, flares, airbags, and munitions. Poor waste management procedures in the manufacturing of perchlorate have allowed the chemical to be released into water systems across the country. Contamination has been confirmed in at least 25 states. Millions of Americans are consuming tap water with highly toxic perchlorate concentrations (4 parts per billion or more). Although insufficient data exists to classify perchlorate as a carcinogen, the chemical should be eliminated from our water supply because it interferes with thyroid function and contributes to a toxic colon.

If you're becoming concerned about the quality of your tap water, purchasing only bottled water might seem like a worthwhile effort. However, studies conducted by the National Resources Defense Council (NRDC) while testing 103 different brands of water determined many brands of bottled water are polluted with contaminants such as synthetic organic chemicals, arsenic, and bacteria.[84]

Insufficient regulation accounts for the shocking amount of bottled water that advertises purity but instead contains contaminants. The NRDC reports "… the FDA's rules completely exempt waters that are packaged and sold within the same state, which account for between 60 and 70 percent of all bottled water sold in the United States … the FDA also exempts carbonated water and seltzer, and fewer than half of the states require carbonated waters to meet their own bottled water standards."[85] **Even bottled waters that have to comply with the FDA are not as rigorously tested for contaminants as tap water in metropolitan areas.**

The council also estimates 25% of the bottled water on the market is actually bottled tap water. Misleading labels fool the public into believing they are drinking pure water when this could not be further from the truth.

Did You Know?

The National Resources Defense Council (NRDC) observed a particular brand of bottle water with mountains and a lake on the label, which advertised its contents as "spring water". The water source for the manufacturing plant was actually a public water line located near a hazardous waste site!

To add insult to injury, studies have found some bottled water also contains C_8, a chemical used to make Teflon®. The toxin was found in southeast Ohio tap water, so residents were given bottled water instead. When the bottled water was tested, traces of C_8 were found—the very chemical they were trying to avoid! Research conducted regarding the safety of plastic bottled water packaging shows that Phlalates and Bisphenols (hormone disruptors and known carcinogens) may be leaching from the plastic used to make the bottles.

Does a Solution Exist?

Of course, there is always a solution for every situation! We know water is essential to digestive and overall health. However, our colons need pure water, and we just can't count on bottled water companies or our government to provide us with clean water. It's up to all of us to do something. Without public outcry, this practice will continue on and on, so please write to your state representatives, city council members, the FDA, and the president. Ask them to support a clean environment by outlawing toxic chemicals in our water and environment.

For pure clean water, my recommendation is to drink distilled water, **Wellness Water®**, (see "Water" in the *Resources* section), or water from a well dug on clean, uncontaminated land. Distilling water involves boiling, evaporating, and then condensing the water, and finally storing it in a sterile container (preferably glass). As the water is boiled, chemicals and other toxins are removed. The drawback of distillation is that important minerals are removed from the water along with the contaminants.

If your goal is temporary detoxification, distilled water works beautifully to help clean out the colon. However, if you regularly consume distilled water, it should be modified to meet your body's nutritional needs. Distilled water can recapture its essential minerals with the addition of a little organic Apple Cider Vinegar. You can do this at home.

How to Make Your Own Toxin-Free Super Water

1. One gallon distilled water, preferably stored in a glass container.

2. Add two to three tablespoons of non-pasteurized organic Apple Cider Vinegar (ACV).

3. Try to drink ½ of your body weight daily in ounces. Example: if you weigh 150 lbs, drink 75 ounces daily.

Distilled water can easily be found at just about any grocery store. Plain ACV can also be found at most stores, but it's often pasteurized which kills the life force of the vinegar. Purchase only non-pasteurized (raw) organic ACV at a natural health food store or purchase it on the Internet.

Raw Apple Cider Vinegar has been used for centuries to remedy many negative health issues. ACV contains vital nutrients the body needs as well as beneficial bacteria that aid in colon function. Raw apple cider vinegar helps regulate pH and reduces the risk of constipation, which in turn reduces your risk of developing a toxic colon.

Regularly drinking distilled or purified water with raw organic ACV can support intestinal health, but this isn't the only thing you can do to prevent unwanted chemicals in water from entering your body. The following chart explains more ways to avoid these dangerous toxins!

How to Eliminate Toxins from Water

- Drink Wellness Water®, clean well water, or distilled water supplemented with raw organic Apple Cider Vinegar.

- Test your water for contaminants with a home water test kit.

- Installing a whole house, water purification unit can eliminate up to 99% of water toxins. If a whole house water purification unit isn't financially feasible, install a lower priced under sink unit in both the bathroom and kitchen.

- Install shower and bath filters—remember your skin absorbs toxins! I recommend the Wellness® shower filter.

- If you have a chlorinated pool, convert it to chlorine free. I use the EcoSmarte™ pool conversion kit, which uses copper ions and ozone.

- The Wellness Carafe™ is a high-quality portable water purifier you can take with you anywhere to purify water.

- When buying bottled water, make sure it is packaged in glass whenever possible.

- Cleanse your colon regularly to prevent the build up of arsenic, fluoride, chlorine, and other water toxins. (See *Chapter 5—The Oxygen Colon Cleanse*).

- Test your water source for arsenic. The PurTest® Arsenic Test is a simple home screening kit for checking water levels for this heavy metal.

- Eat foods that naturally provide sulphur such as garlic, eggs, and onions. Sulphur helps remove arsenic from the body.

- See also "Water Purification" in the *Resources*.

CHAPTER NINE

HOW TO REDUCE INTESTINAL TOXINS FROM DRUGS AND STRESS

Take a few minutes to consider the following scenario: Ms. Jones has been experiencing chronic headaches for weeks. She visits her doctor (a trained professional) for help in getting rid of her pounding pain. "Doctor, I've had a headache for a long time now. It's wearing me down!" "No, problem, Ms. Jones. We'll get you fixed up" he replies. Five minutes later, Ms. Jones walks out of the exam room with a piece of barely legible paper in hand. She drops by the pharmacy on the way home to fill her prescription for pain medication—the standard response.

The pills relieve her headache pain, but a month later, Ms. Jones has to visit her doctor again. "Doctor, I haven't been having regular bowel movements lately and my stomach really hurts." "Oh," he replies, "Did I forget to mention the pain medication can cause constipation and possibly stomach ulcers? Don't worry though. I have something for that as well." Five minutes later, Ms. Jones walks out of the exam room with a new prescription. When she gets home, she takes her pill for headache pain, another pill for constipation, and now one for her stomach trouble.

What's wrong with this picture? First of all, the average time a physician spends with a patient is now less than ten minutes. That's not nearly enough time to diagnose a patient and come up with a treatment plan let alone try to find what the real cause of the pain is! Second, the doctor automatically prescribed a drug without asking any further questions of Ms. Jones or considering any natural alternatives. Medicate it, cut it, or burn it—these seem to be the only options for most medical doctors. If the truth be told, the pain medication probably addressed the pain, but it was really just a quick "band aid" to get Ms. Jones in the office, make her wait an hour or two just to be seen, and then charge her $100.00 for 5 minutes of work.

Let's say you're driving down the highway and the oil light comes on in your car. What are you going to do? Put a piece of tape over the light or smash the dashboard so you can't see it? No, of course not. Hopefully, you'll pull over, look under the hood, and find the source of the problem. If the real problem isn't addressed, all kinds of other mechanical failures can occur. Does your body deserve any less consideration than your car?

The source of Ms. Jones' pain was never addressed. Maybe she was experiencing headaches from drinking too much coffee, maybe she was stressed out from work, she had a bone slightly out of position, or she has an undiagnosed vision problem. The point is—the doctor didn't take the time to find out. He prescribed a medication that masked the headache but damaged the digestive tract as a side effect. Ms. Jones ended up taking three different prescription drugs for a simple headache.

Think about the combined amount of toxic residue from these synthetic pharmaceuticals that's now burdening her body, and it's so unnecessary! It's discouraging to consider how many Americans are taking drugs they don't really need instead of addressing the root cause of their health problems. Obviously, both the medical establishment and the pharmaceutical industry are the only ones benefiting from this strategy. Think about it—when was the last time you heard of any disease or even a common symptom actually being cured?

Staggering Statistics About Modern Medicine and Pharmaceutical Drugs

- Prescription errors (due to ineligible writing) account for millions of deaths every year[86] and occur most often due to simple human error.[87]

- Every year, over 2 million people suffer from adverse drug reactions (ADR's) and other medical errors while in the hospital. Nearly 1 million deaths result from this malpractice annually.[88]

- Every year, up to 20 million people are unnecessarily prescribed antibiotics.[89]

- "The American medical system is the leading cause of death and injury at nearly 800,000 in the US. By contrast, the number of deaths attributable to heart disease in 2001 was 699,697, while the number of deaths attributable to cancer was 553,251."[90]

- "About 1,500 companies in the US manufacture and market medicinal drugs, with combined annual US revenue over $200 billion."[91]

- "US health care spending reached $1.6 trillion in 2003, representing 14% of the nation's gross national product."[92]

- Pharmaceutical companies spent over $39 billion on domestic

> ### Staggering Statistics About Modern Medicine and Pharmaceutical Drugs (contd.)
>
> drug research and development in 2005 alone. Incredibly, this figure represented less than 16% of sales for that same year![93]

Aren't Prescription Drugs Supposed to Fix What's Wrong with You?

Nearly half of all American citizens take at least one prescription drug and about one in five take three or more medications. Pharmaceutical drugs are synthetic, meaning they did not occur in nature but were manufactured. The human body doesn't want synthetic garbage pumped into it. These drugs pollute the body, suppress the immune system, and contribute to colon toxicity. It's heartbreaking to consider that pharmaceuticals have become the quick and easy solution to most health problems. Ironically, most of these "medicines" actually interfere with health. Side effects of common pharmaceuticals include weight gain, constipation, cancer, kidney disease, heart failure, depression, anxiety, chronic pain, and many other ailments they're supposed to remedy.

> **Did You Know?**
>
> The American Medical Association rakes in an additional $20 million annually by selling detailed profiles of all American doctors to pharmaceutical companies. With such information, these companies can market specific drugs directly to physicians in a particular field related to those products' "benefits".

The colon is one of many organs negatively influenced by the routine consumption of prescription drugs. Constipation is a very common

DANGER! These Drugs Cause Constipation!

- Antacids containing aluminum
- Anticonvulsants
- Antidepressants
- Anti-diarrheal agents
- Antihistamines
- Anti-inflammatory agents
- Antipsychotics
- Antispasmodics
- Beta blockers
- Calcium channel blockers
- Decongestants
- Diuretics
- Iron supplements (synthetic)
- Muscle relaxers
- Narcotics (pain relievers)
- Parkinson's Disease drugs
- Sedatives
- Tranquilizers

complaint from people taking certain medications. While many people might believe this is a small price to pay for alleviating their condition, remember that constipation is extremely unhealthy and may cause colorectal cancer if prolonged.

Can Antibiotics Damage My Colon?

Antibiotics are drugs that destroy bacteria or inhibit their growth and are possibly the most over-prescribed medication on Earth. Antibiotics can kill beneficial bacteria, cause diarrhea and colitis, and lead to antibiotic resistance by bacteria if overused. Very commonly, viral infections are misdiagnosed as bacterial infections. In these cases, patients receive a completely pointless dose of antibiotics. **It's estimated that over 50 million pounds of antibiotics are prescribed every year.** In many cases, these drugs are being prescribed needlessly. Whether the prescriptions are necessary or not, these antibiotic drugs are contaminating intestinal tracts and causing serious side effects.

"Good" bacteria (also referred to as friendly bacteria, healthy bacteria, digestive flora, or intestinal flora) take residence in the colon shortly after birth and are passed on through mother's milk. Trillions of these bacteria live, multiply, and help fight off infection. Although a small number of harmful bacteria may be present, they are far outnumbered by the good bacteria keeping them in check. However, antibiotics reduce the number of healthy bacteria, thus allowing the bad bacteria and Candida to thrive.

Clostridium difficile is the most common harmful bacteria that multiply in the colon if antibiotics kill off the friendly bacteria. *Clostridium* produces a toxin that builds up in the colon, causes diarrhea, and severely damages the lining of the colon.

Situations Increasing the Likelihood of Antibiotic-Associated Diarrhea:

- Using antibiotics frequently
- Taking multiple antibiotics for an infection
- Using very powerful antibiotics
- Having a compromised immune system

DOCTOR'S NOTE:
If you have to take antibiotics, use a natural Probiotic formula to replenish the good gut bacteria. I recommend the **Brevibacillus laterosporus B.O.D. strain** *or* **Bacillus coagulans** *(formally known as* **Lactobacillus sporogenes***) to quickly restore bowel health.*

Are Vaccinations Bad for the Colon?

Vaccines have been at the center of debate lately. Although many serious diseases exist, the risk of vaccination side effects outweighs their benefits. These drugs overload the immune system with toxins and depress its function, thereby making the body more susceptible to disease.

Vaccines – The Hidden Poison

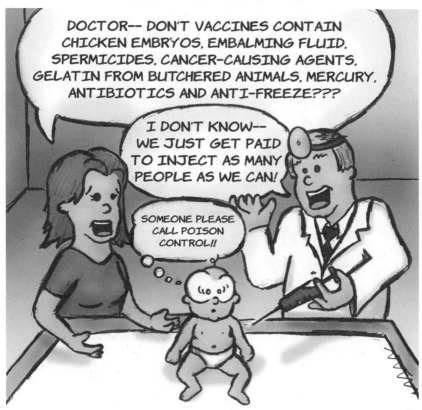

Fig. XI

Do You Know About the True Dangers of Vaccines?

Did your doctor explain the risks to you before he injected you or your child? Many vaccines contain harmful (even lethal) ingredients that damage the colon, blood cells, and other organs in the body. Please do your children a favor and do not vaccinate them! Natural vaccines such as transfer factor, colostrum and Homeopathics are much safer alternatives.

Toxic Ingredients in Common Vaccines

- Chicken embryos (may cause allergic reactions and transmit deadly virus material)

- Living viruses

- Formaldehyde (embalming fluid—a known carcinogen)

- Octoxinol-9 (a spermicidal agent that causes rashes, dizziness, chills, and muscle aches)

- Tritonx-100 (potential carcinogen)

- Foreign DNA and/or RNA fragments from caged lab animals

- Gelatin (made from the boiled skin, tendons, and bones of butchered animals)

- Thimerosal (a derivative of mercury that can result in autism, coma, and death)

- Nonoxynol-9 (a powerful disinfectant and spermicidal ingredient)

- Neomycin, Polymyxin, and Gentamicin (antibiotics)

- Table salt (can cause the gastrointestinal tract to become severely inflamed, along with diarrhea, vomiting, and dehydration)

- Heavy metals such as mercury, aluminum, and a variety of oxides

Pharmaceutical companies don't want you to know about the ingredients (and the damaging effects) in their products. They certainly don't want you to know their drugs overwhelm your body with toxins! With conventional medical doctors in their hip pockets, it's easy for pharmaceutical companies to convince you their products are beneficial. Meanwhile, these companies marginalize or outright attack alternative therapies (such as nutrition, exercise, and natural supplements) so you have no option left but to take their drugs. I want you to know you have other options. Your body belongs to you, not to Big Pharma (a common nickname or euphemism for the collective pharmaceutical industry in the U.S.A.), and you don't have to depend on drugs anymore. Just follow the recommendations in this book and your body can start healing itself once it has been cleansed of toxins.

How to Eliminate Toxins from Prescription Drugs

- Start with information in *Chapter 5—The Oxygen Colon Cleanse* followed by three consecutive Liver/Gallbladder Cleanses, (see *Chapter 12—Dr. Group's Liver and Gallbladder Cleansing, Parasite Cleansing, and Heavy Metal Cleansing*). Drug residue collects in the liver (which should be flushed every six months even if you don't take any drugs). Time-contingent detoxification is a slow process to help wean you off a dependency on medications. Your healthcare provider can help with this phase once you're finished cleansing.

- If drug abuse is an issue, structured intervention may be the best solution. Find a drug rehabilitation center specializing in detoxification and counseling.

- Ask your natural healthcare practitioner about healthful alternatives to drugs.

- Cleanse your colon regularly to help flush toxic pharmaceuticals out of your system and prevent intestinal damage.

- Take Probiotics regularly to replenish the beneficial bacteria in your intestinal tract. (See "Probiotics" in the *Resources* section.)

How Does Stress Affect My Colon?

In today's hectic world, almost no one can escape the effects of stress. Whether it's physical, emotional, or spiritual, stress is responsible for creating or worsening many intestinal ailments. Stress makes the body less capable of protecting itself from disease. The widespread effects of stress are progressively weakening the health of the entire nation. In fact, the American Institute of Stress considers it America's primary health concern.

Staggering Stress Statistics

- Up to 40% of people say their jobs are "... very or extremely stressful."[94]

- "One-fourth of employees view their jobs as the number one stressor in their lives."[95]

- Symptoms of stress can include: headaches, difficulty sleeping, poor concentration, persistent anger, upset stomach (ulcers), lack of digestion, weakened immune system, depression, and overall feelings of dissatisfaction and apathy.[96]

- "Studies show that stressful working conditions are actually associated with increased absenteeism, tardiness, and intentions by workers to quit their jobs-all of which have a negative effect on the bottom line."[97]

- Job stress has been identified as a significant risk factor for a number of health problems, including cardiovascular disease, musculoskeletal disorders, alcoholism/drug addiction, workplace injuries, eating disorders, and even suicide in severe cases.

- It's estimated 3 out of 4 people experience significant levels of stress at least every other week.

Staggering Stress Statistics (contd.)

- "Research indicates that up to one-third of all workers report high levels of stress on the job."[98]

- "48% of workers say they have too much work to do ... and unreasonable deadlines."[99]

- "U.S. workers put in more hours on the job than the labor force of any other industrial nation, where the trend has been just the opposite."[100]

- "An estimated 1 million workers are absent every day due to stress."[101]

What Is Stress?

Stress is subjective. What's stresses one person may be fun or relaxing for another. Only you can understand the limits of your body and mind. Stress has come to have a rather negative connotation in recent years, but we sometimes forget there is good stress as well. Good stress (eustress) results in feelings of excitement or fulfillment and can help someone complete tasks well.

Researchers have found that brief spurts of stress can actually help fortify the immune system. It's the prolonged, bad stress (distress) that you have to worry about. Bad stress manifests as fear, anger, anxiety, or depression.

How Is Stress Related To A Toxic Colon?

Chronic levels of any negative emotion can cause stress hormones (such as corticosteroids) to accelerate or inhibit the movement of waste through the colon. Over time, this can increase one's appetite and lead to unwanted weight gain. The colon is very sensitive to stress responses and its ability to function is easily disrupted by lingering stress.

The Pressures of Modern Education

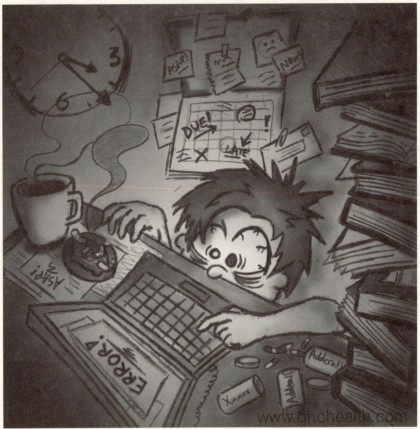

Fig. XII

When people are busy and stressed out, they tend not to take care of their bodies. In the midst of the hustle and bustle of life, many people put off going to the bathroom. Delaying a bowel movement is one of the most common reasons people become constipated. This, in turn leads to a toxic colon. A stressful schedule can also lead many people to eat on the run. Most fast food diets include large portions of meat, fat, sugar, and very little fresh vegetables, whole grains, and water. This type of low fiber diet can lead to both stress and a backed-up colon.

Stressed individuals also skip meals or eat on the go without taking the time to chew their food. Because a regular eating schedule leads to regular bowel movements, inconsistent or rushed meals can likewise lead to problems in the gut and constipation.

Constipation can be a direct result of stress-related changes in the nervous system. Normal bowel movements occur because of complex signals sent by the nervous system. Too much stress causes an interruption of these signals and inhibits intestinal motility, thus resulting in irregular bowel movements.

Amplifying The Effects Of Stress

We've established that bad stress is toxic to the overall health of the colon, but what happens if you add lack of exercise and sleep to the picture? Humans are designed by nature to be on the move, not on the couch. The typical American watches about six hours of television every day and works at a sedentary job. Rarely do people make time to exercise either. It's no surprise the U.S. has become one of the fattest nations in the world.

Exercise powers the lymphatic system. A major role of the lymphatic system is that of waste management. The lymphatic system helps deliver nutrients and remove toxic waste from cells. If the body retains toxins, depression quickly ensues. Remember—depression is one of those negative emotions that can make a person less likely to exercise. So you see, stress is not a single event but a vicious cycle that has to be broken.

The benefits of exercise are not limited to just the lymphatic system. A study published by Texas Tech University reports "… regular exercise reduces the risk of developing colon cancer and the risk of death from colon cancer."[102]

The muscles in the colon benefit from regular exercise as well, and a well-toned digestive tract promotes healthy bowel movements. Lack of exercise causes the muscles surrounding the bowels to weaken and this makes it difficult to fully eliminate waste. Exercise also boosts the immune system which, in turn, helps protect against disease.

Inadequate sleep can also compound the effects of stress and contribute to a toxic colon. Not getting enough sleep at night can disrupt the appetite-regulating hormones and cause people to overeat, which can lead to obesity.

People also tend to make unhealthy dietary choices when they're sleep-deprived. Filling the body with unhealthy food leads to a lack of nutrients to fuel it plus an accumulation of toxins in the colon. Studies indicate sleep deprivation also causes the body to produce more stress hormones, which can cause constipation or aggravate an existing disorder such as Irritable Bowel Syndrome.

Stress Due to Trauma Can Cause Colon Malfunction

Negative emotions can interfere with healthy colon function, but physical stress probably comes to mind first when people think about what wears them down. Trauma (such as pain after an accident or surgery), chronic work-related stress (such as long hours and repetitive or boring work), and especially spinal misalignment can overstress the colon and impair digestive processes. Americans are known for working long hours while most other industrialized countries work fewer hours ... and they are healthier for it!

Did You Know?

America ranks number 28 on a list of developed nations for average life expectancy.[103]

On average, less vacation time is allotted for workers in the United States than almost anywhere else in the industrialized world. Portugal and Spain *require* that workers receive 30 days of vacation annually while Austria, Finland, Sweden, and France each mandate 25 days. However, no amount of vacation time is legally mandated in the United States, so vacation is just an arbitrary period left entirely up to the individual employers! No wonder we're having so many stress-related problems—there's no time for our bodies to regenerate! Basically, physical stress leads to psychological or emotional stress which further compounds the strain on the body and organs such as the colon.

Did You Know A Misaligned Spine Can Cause Colon Dysfunction?

A less obvious physical stressor is a misaligned spine. Injury, poor sitting, sleeping, standing posture, or abnormal growth patterns in the spine result in vertebral misalignment. The displacement of vertebrae is referred to as subluxation, which stresses the spinal muscles, discs, and joints. The nervous system can also become aggravated, which can further hinder organ functions all over the body. The first Lumbar nerve (in the lower back) controls the opening and closing of the ileocecal valve and regulates the contractions of the colon. A misalignment of the L1 vertebrae in the lower back affects the intestinal tract, resulting in possible constipation, diarrhea, or colitis. Hemorrhoids have also been linked to misalignment of the coccyx (tailbone).

⊕ DOCTOR'S NOTE:
A chiropractic spinal realignment can benefit anyone affected by stress, since the nervous system is controlled by spinal impulses. I recommend receiving spinal realignments on a monthly basis. I also recommend spinal exercises to strengthen the muscles supporting the spine.

Common Symptoms of Stress:

- Anger
- Anxiety
- Bossiness
- Compulsive eating
- Constant worry
- Constipation
- Crying often
- Depression
- Excessive alcohol consumption
- Grinding teeth
- Headaches
- Heart palpitations
- Impatience
- Indigestion
- Insomnia
- Irritability
- Muscle aches
- Poor memory
- Sexual dysfunction

Life is demanding and a certain amount of stress is to be expected. Your colon will invariably process some daily toxins due to stress, but chronic levels are debilitating. The body is very sensitive to stress, so

Vertebral Subluxation Chart

Area & Parts of Body	Vertebrae	Possible Effects
Back of Head	**C1**	**C1** - Headaches, Epilepsy, Dizziness
Eyes, Tongue, Forehead	**C2**	**C2** - Allergies, Crossed Eyes, Earache
Cheek, Teeth, Side of Neck	**C3**	**C3** - Acne, Eczema, Neuralgia
Nose, Lips, Mouth	**C4**	**C4** - Hay Fever, Post Nasal Drip
Neck Glands, Vocal Chords	**C5**	**C5** - Laryngitis, Sore Throat
Neck Muscles, Shoulders	**C6**	**C6** - Stiff Neck, Tonsillitis, Croup
Thyroid Gland, Elbows	**C7**	**C7** - Bursitis, Tendinitis, Colds
Hands, Wrists, Fingers	**T1**	**T1** - Carpal Tunnel Syndrome, Asthma
Heart, Coronary Arteries	**T2**	**T2** - Chest Pains, Heart Conditions
Lungs, Bronchial Tubes, Chest	**T3**	**T3** - Bronchitis, Pneumonia, Influenza
Gall Bladder, Common Duct	**T4**	**T4** - Gall Bladder Conditions, Shingles
Liver, Solar Plexus, Blood	**T5**	**T5** - Liver Conditions, Arthritis, Anemia
Stomach, Mid-Back Area	**T6**	**T6** - Indigestion, Heartburn, Dyspepsia
Pancreas, Duodenum	**T7**	**T7** - Diabetes, Ulcers, Gastritis
Spleen, Lower-Mid Back	**T8**	**T8** - Low Back Pain, Infections
Adrenal Glands	**T9**	**T9** - Allergies, Obesity, Hives
Kidneys	**T10**	**T10** - Kidney Trouble, Nephritis
Ureters	**T11**	**T11** - Eczema, Auto-Intoxication
Small Intestines, Upper/Lower Back	**T12**	**T12** - Rheumatism, Gas Pains
Large Intestines, Iliocecal Valve	**L1**	**L1** - Constipation, Colitis, Diarrhea
Appendix, Abdomen, Upper Leg	**L2**	**L2** - Appendicitis, Cramps
Sex Organs, Uterus, Bladder, Knees	**L3**	**L3** - Bladder, Impotence, Knee Pain
Prostate Gland, Lower Back	**L4**	**L4** - Backache, Sciatica, Lumbago
Lower Legs, Ankles, Feet	**L5**	**L5** - Leg Cramps, Swollen Ankles
Hip Bones, Buttocks	**Sacrum**	**Sacrum** - Spinal Curvatures
Rectum, Anus	**Coccyx**	**Coccyx** - Hemorrhoids, Piles, Pruritus

measures must be taken to minimize the overall amount of stress you experience. Review the chart below for living happily and reducing the stress in your life.

How to Eliminate Toxins from Stress

- **The Power of Meditation-** Calming the mind is one of the fastest ways to eliminate stress and negative emotions. Sit quietly, close your eyes, and clear your mind of conscious thought. Sit comfortably, preferably early in the morning and outside in nature. Feel the connection between yourself, the trees, the sky, and the infinite universe. To learn different meditation methods, conduct research online or in a book store to find what works best for you.

- **The Power of Chiropractic-** Receive regular adjustments from a chiropractor to help keep the nerve pathways to the bowels functioning properly and just to relieve stress.

- **The Power of Music-** Music has been documented to help relieve stress, and you can find special CD's for just this purpose. Personally, I recommend the music of Ray Lynch or Robert Aviles.

- **The Power of Exercise-** Exercise increases the production of stress-relieving endorphins. Exercise is a great stress-reliever and has the added benefit of promoting healthy digestion. It may seem like just one more thing to add to your schedule, but exercise is worth it. I recommend rebounding (on a mini trampoline) for stress relief and toxin removal. Plus, it's fun!

- **The Power of Laughter-** Although it might sound corny, look in a mirror and start laughing at yourself. Keep going

How to Eliminate Toxins from Stress (contd.)

and soon you will forget what you were stressed about! Try this with a friend or loved one as well. If you choose to watch TV watch shows that make you laugh!

- **The Power of Massage** - Massage is a great way to relieve tension and relax the body. Try to receive a thorough massage at least once a week. If you cannot afford a massage, touching and hugging relax the body. Hug someone for a few minutes and see how you feel! Or become a tree hugger and hug a tree for 5 minutes. Believe it or not - It WORKS!

- **The Power of Change** – Address what causes your stress and eliminate those factors from your life! If you don't enjoy your life the way it is, make adjustments until you can gradually change things and become the person you want to be. Without change, stressors inside us lie dormant and wait to be released. Resisting the flow of life leads to stagnation.

- **The Power of Sleep** - This is a very important part of your schedule, but most people don't get enough deep restful sleep. If you need help sleeping, I recommend the "Rest Quiet" natural sleep patches.

- **The Power of Nature and the Sun** - If you live in a place where it is convenient to walk in nature, by all means, take advantage of it! However, enjoying just 20 minutes in the sun in your backyard or outside of the office in the morning can energize you. In the evening, exposure to nature can help you unwind and relax. Placing a small waterfall machine in your office or home can help relieve tension by reminding you of nature's calming effects and beauty.

- **The Power of Love** - Create a "Space of Love" for you and your family and cultivate an organic garden to relieve stress. Read the *Anastasia* series of books by Vladimir Megre.

- **The Power of Color** - Dark blue has a calming effect on the body. Try wearing dark blue clothing on days in which you anticipate extra stress.

- **Aromatherapy** - The benefits of aromatherapy date back thousands of years. Stress-relieving essential oils include Lavender, Jasmine, Chamomile, Geranium, Peppermint and Lemongrass. Place a couple of drops in the palm of your hand. Rub your hands together to activate the oils and then cup them together. Deeply inhale the oils through your nose from your cupped hands 8 or 9 times.

- **EFT and NLP** - Emotional Freedom Techniques (EFT) and Neurolinguistic Programming (NLP) are special techniques for helping you relieve stress. Find a practitioner in your area and try them.

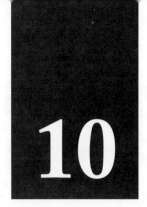

CHAPTER TEN

HOW TO REDUCE INTESTINAL TOXINS FROM HEAVY METALS & RADIATION

Think about the last time you drank a canned beverage, put on deodorant, ate fish, or had a cavity filled at the dentist. Any one of these typical activities potentially exposes the body to toxins from metals. The canned drink and deodorant both contain aluminum, and mercury is a component of dental fillings, and both are extremely toxic metals. Humans and other organisms need very small amounts of the heavy metals zinc, cobalt, manganese, molybdenum, vanadium, copper, and strontium, but even these elements can be damaging to the human body when consumed in excess.

Nonetheless, more than twenty different heavy metals are completely non-essential for human biology. Modern industry has found profitable uses for these toxic elements. The mining and refining of heavy metals has been on the rise ever since.

Did You Know?

Your body can be exposed to toxic metals from cosmetics, medicine, herbal supplements, hygiene products, dental fillings, vaccines, food and beverage storage, cookware, paints, cigarettes, and more.

We're exposed to heavy metal toxins via ingestion, inhalation, and skin or eye contact. Once in the body, heavy metals multiply the production of harmful free radicals (by up to one million times) and cause deadly chain reactions. Heavy metals poison the body, impairing the function of cells, tissues, and organs, and can ultimately lead to cancer and countless other diseases.

Warning! Many herbal supplements have been found to contain levels of heavy metals exceeding federal standards for drinking water by as much as 10 to 20 times! These types of supplements are cheaply made and you will typically find them at drug stores, supermarkets, websites, or discount stores that don't specialize in alternative health. Invest your money on quality health supplements and you'll be investing in your own health at the same time.

Four additional metals that cause damage to the intestinal tract and contribute to colon toxicity are mercury, aluminum, lead, and cadmium. Three of these metals rank in the top 10 on the CERCLA Priority List of Hazardous Substances from the ATSDR.[104] Lead is second, with mercury at a close third, and cadmium falls in as the eighth most toxic substance known to science. Aluminum, although not truly a heavy metal, is still an extremely poisonous substance that can accumulate in the body's tissues. Arsenic, the number 1 most toxic heavy metal, is so prevalent in the public water supply, I focused on it in *Chapter 8—How to Reduce Intestinal Toxins from Air and Water.*

Intestinal Toxins from Mercury

Both organic and inorganic mercury are highly toxic and can cause serious harm to the colon. Inorganic mercury is used in thermometers, thermostats, dental amalgam (fillings), batteries, barometers, skin-tightening creams, various pharmaceutical drugs (e.g. laxatives, diuretics, and antiseptics), and especially medicinal vaccines and pesticides. Inhalation of inorganic mercury vapors is the most common route of exposure, although ingestion, skin contact, and injection are also possible routes.

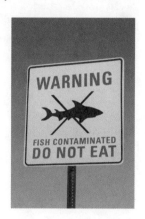

Did You Know?

- *One out of every ten women of childbearing age has dangerously high concentrations of mercury "...within one tenth of potentially hazardous levels" in their bloodstream.*[105]

- *Blue marlin caught in the Gulf of Mexico contain up to 8 times higher mercury levels (over 12 parts per million) than the maximum the EPA allows! "The United States EPA and Florida Department of Health guidelines for fish consumption indicate that any specimen with a mercury level [greater than] 1.5 ppm in their muscle tissue should not be consumed in any amount."*[106]

Organic mercury is usually found in fish and other aquatic organisms but can also be detected in produce, livestock, processed grains, and dairy products. Most commonly, humans are exposed to mercury by eating contaminated fish or inhaling fumes from dental fillings. Refer to the following table for avoiding mercury found in fish. Avoid eating fish in the Danger and Caution Zones!

Organic Mercury Concentration in Commercial Fish

MODERATE ZONE
(Lowest Concentration)

- Anchovies
- Butterfish
- Carp
- Catfish
- Clam
- Cod
- Crawfish
- Croaker (Atlantic)
- Haddock (Atlantic)
- Herring
- Mackerel Atlantic (North Atlantic)

- Mackerel Chub (Pacific)
- Monkfish
- Mullet
- Oyster
- Perch
- Salmon
- Sardine
- Scallop
- Squid
- Tilapia
- Trout (freshwater)
- Whitefish

CAUTION ZONE
(Medium Concentration)

- Bass (Chilean, Saltwater, Black, Striped)
- Bluefish

- Sablefish
- Scorpionfish

- Buffalofish
- Grouper (all species)
- Halibut
- Lobster (Northern, American)
- Mackerel Spanish (Gulf of Mexico)
- Marlin
- Orange Roughy
- Sea Trout
- Sheepshead
- Skate
- Snapper
- Tilefish (Atlantic)
- Tuna (all species)
- White Croaker (Pacific)

DANGER ZONE
(Highest Concentration)

- King Mackerel
- Shark
- Swordfish
- Tilefish (Gulf of Mexico)

The degree of poisoning depends on the form of mercury consumed. Inorganic forms of mercury are usually considered more toxic than organic forms since they possess highly corrosive properties. On the bright side, inorganic mercury cannot be fully absorbed by the intestinal tract. Organic mercury, on the other hand, can be absorbed all too readily. Certain forms of organic mercury also convert into inorganic compounds. This conversion significantly increases its toxicity, causing its effects on the colon to become similar to those of inorganic mercury.

✚ DOCTOR'S NOTE:
Gastrointestinal symptoms of mercury exposure include abdominal cramps, vomiting, diarrhea, constipation, bloating, excessive gas, loss of appetite, obesity, and hemorrhage.

The use of mercury amalgam fillings for tooth cavities has generated renewed concern about this toxin. Once these fillings are in place, they continue to emit mercury vapors into the foods you eat. Once swallowed, these mercury particles end up in your intestinal tract. In fact, mercury's toxicity is so potent that walking into a typical dentist's office can expose an individual to the same amount of mercury (as fumes) as 19 amalgam fillings! The only "safe" amount of mercury in the body is none!

Did You Know?

- Many people have developed colitis from chronic ingestion of mercury-containing laxatives.

- Many common vaccines contain Thimerosal (nearly 50% mercury in structure) to preserve their ingredients.

Intestinal Toxins from Aluminum

As mentioned before, aluminum isn't actually a heavy metal, but I've chosen to include it since it can be found in so many modern products. The prevalence of aluminum and aluminum alloys in such a wide variety of items is especially troubling because it's toxic even in small amounts. Ever since refining developments in the 1880s permitted inexpensive extraction of the metal, more and more products containing aluminum have been introduced to consumers. In my opinion, this rampant mercury usage has gotten out of hand. Review the following table for some of the most common products manufactured with aluminum.

Mercury Dental Filling Vapors

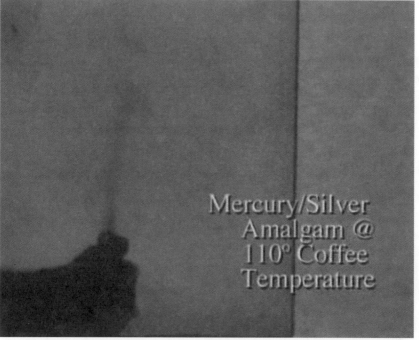

Fig. XIII: Mercury filling vapors photographed with special equipment

Warning! These Products May Contain Aluminum!

- Antacids
- Anti-diarrhea medication
- Antiperspirants
- Astringents
- Baking powder
- Buffered aspirin

- Cans (food and drink)
- Cookware
- Dentures
- Fireworks
- Foil
- Hemorrhoid medications

- Lipstick
- Nasal sprays
- Processed cheese
- Toothpaste
- Vaccines
- Vaginal douches

The average individual frequently "consumes" or uses multiple items on that list every day. Try to find an urban household without any aluminum cans, foil, baking powder, or aspirin. Sadly, manufactured goods are not the only source of aluminum exposure. Increased levels of acid rain infuse dissolved aluminum compounds into the earth, and this has led to the deposit of these toxins in both fresh and salt water. Previously clean sources of drinking water have now been polluted plus countless marine species have been contaminated by the after-effects of our "disposable" culture.

Aluminum can be absorbed either through the intestinal tract or the lungs depending on the point of initial exposure. Drinking soda from a can, for example, dumps aluminum toxins into the intestinal tract. The aluminum is slowly absorbed and can wind up in other bodily tissues. Alzheimer's, Parkinson's disease and many other nervous system disorders are now being linked to excess aluminum deposited in the delicate brain tissue.

Ingestion of foods heated in aluminum cookware is also believed to contribute to inflammation of the digestive tract. Moderate use of antacids has been linked to health problems, as many of these medicines contain aluminum hydroxide—a toxic compound. Aluminum hydroxide stresses the digestive system and can disrupt healthy bowel function. Can you believe the FDA fights every day to limit your access to natural health supplements yet approves literally thousands of these poisonous products for sale?

Intestinal Toxins from Lead

Lead is the second most hazardous substance according to the ATSDR (Agency for Toxic Substances and Disease Registry).[107] Lead is a soft metal used in paints, pipes, drains, and soldering equipment. These practices have largely been abandoned, but we can still find lead in many products due to outright disregard for human safety.

Products Potentially Containing Lead

- Ammunition (powder)
- Antiques (due to coatings, paints, etc.)
- Batteries (especially for autos)
- Cable coverings
- Ceramics
- Cigarettes
- Crystal and glass (especially Depression-era)
- Fuel
- Paints (foreign or cheap grades mostly)
- Pesticides
- PVC plastics
- Weights
- X-ray shields
- Toys and products imported from China and other countries.

Products intentionally manufactured with lead aren't the only concern. Lead exposure most often occurs when airborne particulates and paints containing lead contaminate drinking water. This is due partly to lead-filled fumes from mining, smelting, and manufacturing processes, as well as the inadequate removal of toxic lead-based paints. These airborne lead particles drift to the ground after a week or so, and pollute the soil and water sources. Drinking water can be contaminated in this manner, or from traveling through lead-based plumbing materials. Pipes, for example, can become corroded, resulting in higher concentrations of lead in the water. Many homes built before 1940 are danger zones, especially if lead pipes haven't been replaced and the walls were painted with lead-based paints. Tobacco smoke can also contain dangerous amounts of lead. People who smoke or who are exposed to secondhand smoke are prime candidates for lead poisoning.

Lead poisoning can occur from inhaling or ingesting the toxic metal. Around 90% of lead inhaled into the lungs is absorbed directly into the bloodstream. Most of it is absorbed into the bones, but some lead makes its way to soft tissues and organs. Ingested lead is first broken down in the stomach and then absorbed into the blood through the intestinal lining. From this point, ingested lead travels to organs and organ systems. Lead poisons the body and results in a number of symptoms, including abdominal pain and constipation. Recently, multiple retailers were forced to recall million of toys made in China due to high levels of lead. Could China be secretly disposing of their hazardous waste by hiding it in the products they ship overseas?

Intestinal Toxins from Cadmium

In general, people are not as aware of the dangers of cadmium as they are of metals such as arsenic, mercury, aluminum, and lead. Cadmium is an extremely toxic heavy metal even in small quantities. Since it's poorly excreted, cadmium can collect slowly in intestinal and body tissue. Over time, damage to the intestines can result and digestion may be severely disrupted.

An article in *Toxicology* reported that mice administered a single dose of cadmium (by mouth) developed gastroenteritis (irritation and inflammation of the stomach and intestines).[108] Just one dose! This is scary considering many humans are exposed to cadmium multiple times a day, especially if they smoke or are subjected to cigarette smoke. Smoking just one cigarette introduces the body to around 20 micrograms! Only half of this is excreted, meaning about 10 micrograms remain in other parts of the body.

Consumption of contaminated food products can also expose the body to the poisonous effects of cadmium. Many industrial operations expel cadmium compounds into the environment which wind up in edible crops as well as animal meat and milk. Consuming foods and beverages contaminated with cadmium over prolonged periods can result in serious intestinal problems such as colon cancer. For example, some teas and coffee contain cadmium so it's best to stick to organic brands whenever possible. Refer to the chart below for additional foods that may contain this toxin.

Foods That May Contain Cadmium

Food	Common Levels (parts per million)
1. Shelled seeds	0.48
2. Organ meats (liver and kidney)	0.15
3. Cabbage	0.1·1
4. Potato Chips	0.10
5. Peanut butter and peanuts	0.07
6. French fries	0.06
7. Cookies	0.06
8. Celery	0.06
9. Cereals (wheat and bran)	0.05
10. Potatoes (boiled with the skin on)	0.04

How Can I Protect Myself from Toxic Heavy Metals?

Every day your colon has to deal with these and other hazardous metals. Dangerous heavy metals and their compounds must be eliminated from the colon to help restore proper digestive function. Detoxifying the body, coupled with an active effort to avoid sources of heavy metal exposure, is a big step in the right direction. The recommendations below are essential in cleansing the body and intestinal tract of toxic heavy metals.

How to Eliminate Toxins from Heavy Metals

- Get tested for heavy metals. Many chiropractors or natural healthcare practitioners can perform this test for you, either through hair, blood, or urine analysis.

- Use FIR therapy. Far Infrared Therapy (FIR), also known as heat therapy, dissolves toxins in the blood so you can sweat them out. Remember, the skin is the largest detoxification organ. If you can afford a Far Infrared Sauna (up to $3000.00), I highly recommend them. FIR helps the body re move heavy metals, aids digestion, and relieves stress. I recommend the brand TheraSauna™.

- Have your mercury amalgams removed ASAP since dental fillings produce vapors which leak into your body. Find a biological dentist who has experience in removing mercury fillings.

- Use ion foot baths. These devices work by delivering an electric current into the body through the feet. Charged ions attach to heavy metal toxins and neutralize them. The metals are then pulled out of the body through your feet as you soak them.

- Eliminate your exposure to aluminum! Use natural antiperspirant that does not contain aluminum. Replace aluminum cookware with silicone bake ware and utensils, Le Creuset®, Range Kleen, cast iron, surgical stainless steel, or lead-glaze free terra cotta. Avoid drinking beverages in aluminum cans also.

- Cleanse your body of toxins. Perform an intestinal cleanse (see *Chapter 5—The Oxygen Colon Cleanse*) plus 3 consecutive liver and gallbladder cleanses (see *Chapter 12— Liver, Gallbladder, Parasite and Heavy Metal Cleansing*) to flush out stored toxic metals from your system.

- Consume only fish with the lowest possible levels of mercury. See the table *Organic Mercury Concentration in Commercial Fish* in this chapter.

- Don't allow anyone to give you a vaccination! Please save yourself and your children from the harmful effects of vaccinations such as the heavily marketed flu shot. Vaccines are extremely toxic, contaminated with a variety of known poisons (by design), and largely unnecessary. Why would anyone still need to receive vaccines for diseases that haven't been common for decades?

- See "Cookware", "Heat Therapy", "Heavy Metals", and "Ion Foot Baths" in the *Resources* section.

Eliminating Intestinal Toxins from Radiation

Is radiation harmful to humans? Normally, you can't see it, smell it, taste it, hear it, or feel it, so what's so bad about it? Even though radiation is intangible, its a very real danger. Typically, radiation seems to be a threat only in the context of large-scale events (e.g. nuclear bomb blasts) that produce enough radiation to damage or destroy body tissues immediately. However, the effects of long-term exposure to low-level radiation can be just as deadly. Electromagnetic radiation is simply energy emitted in the form of particles or waves. This section will focus mainly on harmful electromagnetic field radiation (EMF) as you would encounter from common devices and machines generating electrical currents.

Power lines, cellphones, computers, transformers, fluorescent lights, clock radios, and even hair dryers are just a few of the modern devices that emit dangerous electromagnetic waves. In addition to artificial sources of radiation, fault lines under the ground are natural sources of potentially harmful radiation as well.

When electromagnetic radiation comes into contact with living matter, it causes ionization—the loss of electrons from atoms. This process negatively affects DNA, and can result in chromosomal mutation or even cellular damage and death. If losing electrons negatively affects a cell, then it can also affect tissue, which will affect organs, and then entire bodily systems. You can see where I'm going with this. Basically, you don't want to lose electrons.

Unfortunately, in our modern world, losing electrons is much easier than gaining them. Watching TV, talking on cellular devices, working in an office with fluorescent lights—all these activities expose you to EMF's and can cause your body to lose electrons. The body needs electrons to remain healthy. You can regain electrons by walking in the woods or along the beach, breathing pure oxygen, and eating live fruits and vegetables. These activities contribute electrons to your body to help it regenerate. Without a doubt, most Americans do nothing to counteract the effects of electron-stealing radiation and they also saturate themselves with harmful EMF's by surrounding themselves with all the latest trendy gadgets, toys, technology, and other trivial "conveniences".

You might be thinking, "Hey, a little radiation when I use the Internet, watch TV, or talk on my cellphone won't hurt. It really doesn't matter. It's not like I'm sticking my head in the microwave oven." Well, guess what—it does matter! If you ingest a teaspoon of salt 100 times a day, it's going to add up.

John Gofman, professor emeritus of Medical Physics at UC Berkeley and an expert on radiation's health effects, is one of the most outspoken forces against unnecessary exposure to radiation. He states, "There is no safe threshold. If this truth is known, then any permitted radiation is a permit to commit murder." [109] Dr. Gofman certainly knows what he's talking about since he helped produce plutonium for the Manhattan Project, which was the United States' top secret program for developing the first atomic bombs. All of those seemingly insignificant interactions with electrical devices add up over time. These daily, low doses of radiation increase your risk of developing several cancers including colon cancer. Radiation overstresses the colon and disrupts digestive processes, leading to abdominal pain, constipation, diarrhea, and cancer.

We're literally swimming in radiation every day. Urban areas in particular bombard the human body with toxic EMF's at home, work, school, and even outdoors. Although some exposure is inevitable, it really has gotten out of hand. Let's examine harmful sources of radiation affecting us on a daily basis.

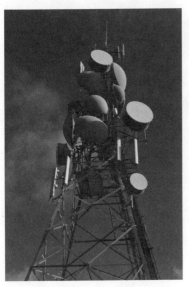

Toxic EMF's from Cellphones and Cellular Towers

Wireless phones are advertised as the ultimate modern convenience, and the ability to communicate on the go is not something people want to give up easily. However, frequent and prolonged use of cellphones can result in very serious health complications, such as brain tumors and cellular damage.

The image on the following page is the head of a man exposed to cellphone radiation for 15 minutes. The man held the cellphone on his left ear. The dark grey area represents the high levels of radiation emitted by the cellphone.

The Swedish National Institute for Working Life, in collaboration with the University of Oerebro, discovered that heavy users of cellphones display "... a 240 percent increased risk for a malignant tumor on the side of the head where they typically held the phone".[110] You might think the effects of mobile phones are limited to just the facial and cranial areas, but that's not always the case. **A report submitted to the Economic Union in 2000**

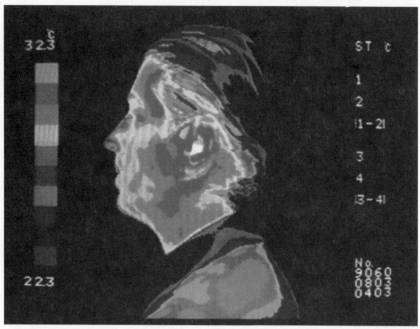

Fig.XIV: Cellphone radiation after only 15 minutes captured with spectrographic X-Ray. Darker areas represent higher levels of radiation.

found that three members of a surveillance unit of the Royal Ulster Constabulary all contracted and died from colon cancer. The members routinely carried radio frequency (RF) transmitters near their lower backs during service.[111] Guess what? RF radiation is exactly what is emitted from cellular phones!

Wearing a cellphone on a clip at your waist or keeping it in your pocket can present serious consequences since the intestinal tract is highly sensitive to radiation. Even the U.S. Department of Labor recognizes that RF radiation (as well as microwave radiation) can heat and damage bodily tissues and it warns against extensive use of cellphones. **A report conducted by the National Council on Radiation Protection and Measurements concludes that human colon cancer cells can become even more cancerous if exposed to low frequency radiation (such as that from a mobile phone).**[112]

An article in *Occupational Medicine* suggests diseases such as Thyroiditis and Inflammatory Bowel Disease can be initiated by low frequency electromagnetic fields (50 Hz).[113] This radiation may compromise the intestinal mucosa, irritate the colon, and contribute to ongoing inflammation.

Did You Know?

Over 1 billion people worldwide own cellular devices, unknowingly subjecting their bodies to the damaging effects of RF radiation. On average, people spend 8 hours or more a month using their cellular device.

Despite the presence of numerous studies indicating the overwhelming health risks of cellphone overuse, wireless industry representatives met at the Institute of Electrical and Electronics Engineers in 1999 and unanimously approved to raise the radiation exposure limit (for increased "range" and "reception" of course). Obviously, wireless companies want to protect their interests and they consistently cover-up the documented scientific evidence implicating the serious health risks of their products. It amazes me what some people will do for money. The sad part is that all they would need to do is place a small, frequency-absorbing chip in each phone and we would be protected.

Unbelievably, a national wireless company (Cingular™) tried to modify their customer contract by including fine print preventing consumers from participating in class-action lawsuits. However, the 9th U.S. Circuit Court of Appeals quickly overruled the fraudulent and "illegal" stipulation.[114]

Similarly, U.S. Senate Bill S.800 was authored "…to encourage and facilitate the prompt deployment throughout the United States of a seamless, ubiquitous, and reliable end-to-end infrastructure for communications, including wireless communications, to meet the Nation's public safety and other communications needs."[115] The bill, while being touted

The Modern Skyline of Disease

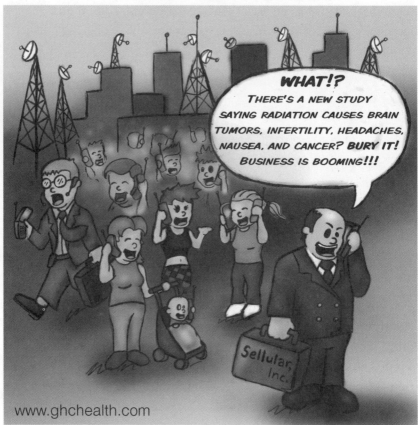

Fig. XV

to enhance "public safety", also has sections tacked on to grant immunity to cellphone manufacturers and vendors for any liability related to their products. Specifically, "any wireless provider, its officers, directors, employees, vendors, and agents, shall have immunity or other protection from liability …."[116] Wireless companies are also protected in that insurance companies will not pay out for illnesses caused by prolonged low frequency radiation exposure! I think we should be asking, what is so special about cellular service providers that they should be permitted to continuously market harmful products while simultaneously being protected from prosecution under established law? That's like committing murder legally with no repercussion.

Well, as usual, there's another radiation culprit to consider. The antennae on top of cellular base towers emit RF radiation at extremely high power. Sometimes, cell antennae are installed on rooftops or the sides of buildings instead of towers in exchange for monetary compensation to the building owners. At these locations, the amount of radiated power can exceed guidelines posted by the Federal Communications Commission (FCC) and can cause harm to anyone in proximity to the antennae. Does the building you work in have cellphone antennae? These building owners are getting rich for permitting the installation and operation of toxic radiation-emitting equipment at the expense of your health!

Toxic Radiation from Home Electronics

Many common household devices, as convenient or entertaining as they may be, also emit harmful radiation. The combined effect of using various electronic devices can seriously damage the ultra-sensitive colon. Keep in mind the typical guideline for safe exposure is between 0.5 and 2 milligauss of radiation; but many household devices emit EMF's in excess of this safety guideline. The greater the field generated, the higher the risk to your health.

Even some non-electronic items can increase the effects of radiation absorbed from another source. Wire-support undergarments, for instance, can behave like antennae and direct EMF's straight into breast tissue. By concentrating the dose of radiation received while wearing some types of bras, you can actually increase your likelihood of developing breast cancer. Beds with metal frames and/or springs can be magnetized by nearby electrical devices (if the field is strong enough) and disrupt bodily functions during sleep.

In addition to the dangers of EMF radiation lurking in the home environment, certain jobs have been linked to excessive exposure. In just one workday, tons of industries expose their employees to dangerous amounts of radiation. The following chart outlines which workers are at the highest risk for developing health problems and the potential amount of radiation they are exposed to every day.

Daily Occupational Exposure to EMF Radiation

Occupation	Typical Exposure (in milligaus)
Cable splicers	Up to 15 mG
Distribution substation operators	Up to 34 mG
Electricians	Up to 34 mG
Line workers	Up to 35 mG
Machinists	Up to 28 mG
TV repair workers	Up to 8 mG
Welders	Up to 96 mG

Remember: Safe Exposure levels are .5 to 2 milligaus

Exposure to high levels of EMF radiation, day after day, slowly causes colon function to deteriorate. Johns Hopkins University has found that workers who splice telephone cables run a higher risk of developing colon cancer. Cable splicers can be exposed to upwards of 15 mG every day. If someone runs a greater risk for colon cancer with only 15 mG, think about the implications for machinists, substation operators, electricians, line workers, and welders. Anyone with one of these occupations could be exposed to at least 28 mG of EMF radiation every day!

Even if you work in an office, you're not safe from the corruptive effects of EMF rays. Many offices use fluorescent lighting which has been linked to a wide range of symptoms and illnesses.

 DOCTOR'S NOTE:
Researchers have found that exposure to fluorescent lights at night disrupts

the body's **circadian rhythm** and a study conducted in 1986 found that fluorescent lighting can increase the likelihood of developing certain cancers.[117] This is especially troubling for anyone (such as employees of most offices, hospitals, retail stores, and restaurants) that have to work for extended periods every day under this type of lighting. Exposure to fluorescent lights has also been linked to an increase in stress hormones. Remember—stress hormones disrupt healthy bowel function and contribute to a toxic intestinal environment!

> **DEFINITION**
>
> *Circadian Rhythm:* The internal biorhythms of living things that are finely attuned to the changing days, seasons, and environmental.

Toxic Effects Of Geopathic Stress

Geopathic stress is produced by a disturbance of the earth's natural electromagnetic field. Underground water, mineral concentrations, tunnels, and fault lines distort the natural frequencies of the earth's field. Plants, animals, and humans living in areas where radiation emanates from the earth are described as being "geopathically stressed" (GS). This condition makes people more susceptible to the development of a variety of emotional and physical problems. Dulwich Health has diagnosed over 40,000 people "…with most types of serious and long term illnesses" and they believe geopathic stress contributes greatly to these individuals' illnesses.[118]

Do you experience unexplained fatigue, depression, anxiety, insomnia, restlessness, nightmares, teeth grinding, "pins and needles" in your arms or legs, headaches, or sleep walking? If conventional treatments have failed, you might be suffering from geopathic stress (GS).

Did You Know?
It's estimated 85% of people with poor health are sleeping in an area affected by geopathic stress (GS).

Sleeping at night in an area that's geopathically stressed is especially dangerous since negative radiation is stronger at night and approximately one-third of your life is spent sleeping.

How Do I Protect Myself from Radiation?

As I mentioned before, exposure to a little radiation is unavoidable. For better or worse, modern society relies on electronics. If we want to keep all these gadgets and live wherever we want, we'll just have to protect ourselves as much as we can from cellular towers, fault lines, and underground sources emitting negative radiation. We can take measures to limit the amount of daily electromagnetic radiation to which we and our loved ones are exposed. By following the recommendations in the chart below, I believe you can reduce your daily radiation exposure by up to 80%.

How to Reduce Toxins from Radiation

- When using a cellphone, use the speaker or an extension with an earpiece instead of holding the phone next to your head.

- Carry the phone in a bag away from the body, but not in your pocket or on a belt-clip.

- Everyone should have an EMF protection device on his or her cellphone. I use the Safe Space™ brand.

- Turn off electronics such as TV's and computers when not in use. Try not to sit too close to appliances and limit the amount of time you use them. This can drastically reduce EMF exposure.

- For your home and office, use a Safe Space™ Clearing Device to clear up to 1500 square feet of harmful radiation.

- Replace all fluorescent lighting and standard light bulbs in your home and office with Full Spectrum or LED lighting.

- For clearing geopathic stress, I highly recommend the Safe Space™ 3—an imprinted holographic 20-inch copper tube intended to reduce energy fluctuations around your home. The tube can be buried in the ground near your house to neutralize a 200-acre area of Geopathic Stress.

- Ladies of all ages should not wear wire bras or other wire-framed garments.

- Use a detector such as the (Radalert™ 100) to check the levels of radiation in your home and workplace.

- Take a proactive stance and write the cell phone company CEOs and the local and federal government asking them for more testing and protection from these harmful devices.

- See "Radiation", "Fluorescent Lighting", and "Geopathic Stress" in the *Resources*.

How to Eliminate or Reduce EMF Radiation from Home Electronics

(Safe exposure levels are between 0.5 and 2 milligauss of radiation daily.)

Household Electronic	Typical Exposure
1. Hair dryer - The motor emits high levels of EMF's close to the handle. Wearing metal hair clips can increase the amount of radiation absorbed. Reduce radiation by drying your hair naturally or place a Safe Space™ EMF protection device on the handle.	Emits up to 70 milligauss
2. Clock radio - The field of radiation is greater with an electro-mechanical clock than it is with an electronic/digital clock. Reduce radiation by using battery-powered clocks or place the clock 6 feet away from your bed.	Emits up to 6 milligauss
3. Computer monitor - Attach an EMF protection device to your laptop and/or desktop computer. This can reduce up to 90% of the radiation from these devices. Never use a	Emits up to 134 milligauss

laptop on your lap as this can promote cervical, ovarian, prostate, and testicular cancer.

4. Electric kettle - Using electricity to boil water changes the structure of its molecules and can cause adverse reactions in many people. Boil water on the range using only non-toxic cookware.	Emits up to 10 milligauss
5. Television - Sitting too close (within 6 feet) to the television exposes the body to high levels of EMF's. Place a Safe Space™ clearing device in the room with the TV you use most commonly. Reduce TV and video game time to 2 hours daily if possible. Spend more time enjoying nature instead of watching TV.	Emits up to 13 milligauss
6. Electric can opener - Unbelievably, this is one of the riskiest devices as it emits an extremely high field of radiation. Throw your electric can opener away and replace it with a handheld opener. Reduce or eliminate eating canned foods, not only for this reason, but	Emits up to 163 milligauss

How to Eliminate or Reduce EMF Radiation from Home Electronics (contd.)

(Safe exposure levels are between 0.5 and 2 milligauss of radiation daily.)

Household Electronic	Typical Exposure
because they can contaminate the food inside.	
7. Microwave oven - Close proximity to a microwave can damage sensitive bodily tissues. Get the microwave out of your house as soon as possible. They are extremely toxic to you and they literally "nuke" foods free of nutrients.	Emits up to 54 milligauss
8. Electric shaver/razor - The design of this device requires skin contact near the teeth. These devices emit 100 milligauss of radiation at a distance of less than 6 inches. Think of the possible increase in EMF levels as the shaver makes contact with your skin at 0 inches! Do you suffer from gingivitis, tooth decay, or chronic oral problems? Your shaver could be the culprit. Trust an old-fashioned razorblade system	Emits up to 100 milligauss

to give you the best shave. And with no EMF's.

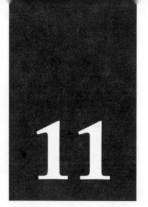

CHAPTER ELEVEN

HOW TO REDUCE INTESTINAL TOXINS FROM PARASITES

Unfortunately, the colon provides a welcoming environment for dangerous invaders such as bacteria, viruses, yeasts, and worms. These invading organisms can enter the human body through air, soil, food, and water. Their interaction with a human host can be unpleasant (and let's face it, pretty gross). I simply must address the threat of hostile organisms (parasites). Everyone is affected by parasites at some point—this is one of the most overlooked health problems facing humanity. Just ridding your body of parasites can boost your energy levels and overall sense of wellbeing.

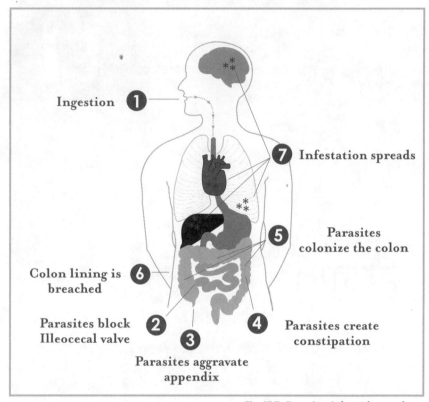

Fig. XVI: Parasites infest a human host

Intestinal Parasites

Many people associate parasitic infestation with less developed nations that may have lower standards for food preparation or personal hygiene. However, parasites pose a very large and very real threat throughout the industrialized world. In fact, parasites are almost as common in the United States and Western Europe as they are anywhere else. If you think you can't possibly become infected with a parasite, consider this—experts estimate up to 3 out of 5 people may have parasites in their bodies and don't even know it![119]

Most people associate the word "parasite" with worms. This is not necessarily so. By definition, parasites are organisms that live on or inside another organism called a "host." These particular invaders can range from microscopic amoebas, bacteria, fungi, and viruses to large intestinal worms measuring several feet in length. These lifeforms operate on pure survival instinct, competing with you for nutrients and excreting toxic waste that can threaten your health. In addition, parasites can cause further damage throughout the host's body as they migrate and encase themselves in hard protective shells in search of food and welcoming environments.

Parasitic infestation can mimic the symptoms of an estimated 50 different diseases. In my personal opinion, I believe parasites are the root cause of many common health conditions.

Symptoms of Parasitic Infection

- Abdominal pain
- Allergies
- Anemia
- Chronically weakened immune system
- Colon cancer
- Constipation
- Dermatitis
- Diarrhea
- Excess gas
- Chronic Fatigue
- Irritable Bowel Syndrome
- Joint Inflammation
- Muscle pain
- Nervousness
- Sleeping problems
- Teeth grinding
- Weight loss

Parasites can be particularly dangerous to the health of the intestinal tract as they not only steal vital nutrients from the body and destroy the colon's permeability, but they also emit harmful toxins in the form of waste. In this chapter, I will cover the most common parasites specific to

> **DEFINITION**
>
> *Lipids:*
> Any hydrophobic (repelled by water) molecule, such as fatty acids and cholesterol, found in living organisms. Lipids can include triglycerides, phospholipids, and metabolites to name a few.

the intestinal tract and liver. **Harmful invaders can include Giardia, Toxoplasma, Cyclospora, Tapeworms, Roundworms/Pinworms, Hookworms, Trichinella, Intestinal fluke, Liver fluke, Candida, E-Coli, Clostridium, and Salmonella.**

✚ DOCTOR'S NOTE:
I will provide methods for eliminating these harmful organisms in Chapter 12 under the section for Parasite Cleansing.

Giardia lamblia (*Giardia intestinalis*)

Picture a microscopic view of your small intestine with millions of these creatures swimming around. I think that would gross anyone out!

Giardia lamblia is a protozoan that lives in the intestinal tract and causes an infection known as Giardiasis. Protective cysts form around the parasite and their eggs. These cysts interfere with your body's digestion of **lipids** and prevent important fat-soluble nutrients from being absorbed. Giardia lamblia ranks as the most common intestinal parasite and reason for diarrhea in the United States and also infects "… approximately 2% of the adults and 6 to 8% of the children in developed countries worldwide."[120] Giardia cysts are passed through feces and can survive for several months even without a host. These organisms then wait for a new host to ingest them through a contaminated source (such as food and water) or through contact with fecal matter. Symptoms of infection include severe diarrhea, bloating, gas, abdominal cramping, weight loss, greasy bowel movements, and dehydration.

Daycare centers are commonly associated with exposure to Giardia and other pathogens. In fact "19% of the clinic visits for acute diarrhea were attributable to child care, with the odds of infection being up to 3 times higher than in non-communal settings!"[121] This parasite is associated with a quarter of all cases of gastrointestinal illness and is not always easily detected. Daycare workers, international travelers, anyone swimming in rivers, lakes, and steams, and people who inadvertently drink water from contaminated sources are easy targets for Giardia be-

Giardia Infestation

ANATOMICAL OVERVIEW:

Typical sites within the small intestine for Giardia lamblia infestation.

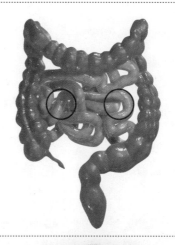

INTERIOR VIEW:

Colonization occurs with adult organisms feeding off the host and reproducing.

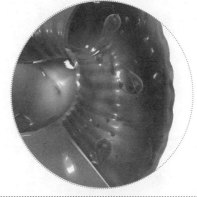

MAGNIFIED VIEW:

Protective cyst encasing a parasite "family" with adult organisms and their eggs.

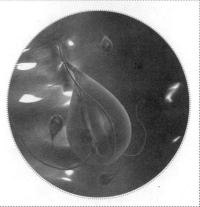

Fig. XVII

cause untreated water is a haven for this parasite.

> **Did You Know?**
>
> *Giardiasis is also referred to as "beaver fever" due to the high rate of infection among campers. Such naturalists may drink water contaminated with beaver droppings containing Giardia.*

Toxoplasma gondii

The Toxoplasma parasite is a single-celled organism that can make its home in the intestinal tract and cause toxoplasmosis. People are usually infected after eating contaminated meat, but they can also contract the parasite by coming into contact with cat feces while gardening or cleaning a litter box. A pregnant woman who is infected with toxoplasmosis can pass the disease to her unborn child who may then develop a central nervous system disorder, spleen or liver enlargement, heart or eye damage, or even mental retardation.

Based on a simple review of available data, over 47 million people living in the U.S.A. may host the Toxoplasma parasite.[122] Healthy individuals with uncompromised immune systems often show no symptoms, but those with weakened immune systems can suffer greatly from this parasite.

Cyclospora cayetanensis

Cyclospora cayetanensis is another common parasitic protozoan that can infect the bowels. Infection occurs from contaminated food and water and from contact with fecal matter. Symptoms include diarrhea, loss of appetite, weight loss, bloating, gas, stomach pain, nausea, vomiting, muscle aches, fever, and fatigue. Once inside the body, Cyclospora parasites invade the intestinal tract where they mature and multiply at an exponential rate. Eventually, the eggs of the parasite are excreted in the waste of the host to begin a new cycle. See image on page 270.

Toxoplasma Infestation

ANATOMICAL OVERVIEW:

Typical sites within the small intestine for Toxoplasma infestation.

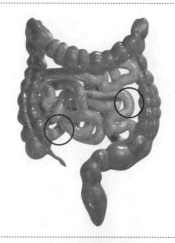

INTERIOR VIEW:

Colonization occurs with adult organisms creating a health condition known as toxoplasmosis.

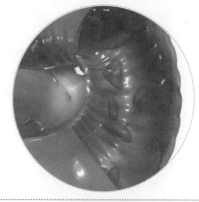

MAGNIFIED VIEW:

Protective cyst encasing a parasite "family" with adult organisms and their eggs.

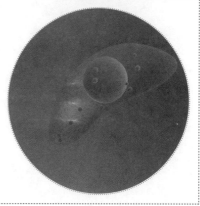

Fig. XVIII

Cyclospora Infestation

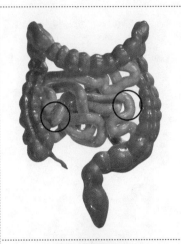

ANATOMICAL OVERVIEW:

Typical sites within the small intestines for Cyclospora infestation.

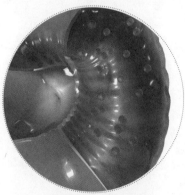

INTERIOR VIEW:

Colonization by adult organisms occurs rapidly due to multiple, asexual reproductive cycles.

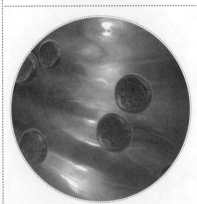

MAGNIFIED VIEW:

A single Cyclospora protozoan can lead to full colonization and severe illness.

Fig. XIX

Parasitic Worms That Can Invade the Colon

Tapeworms

> **DEFINITION**
>
> **Cysticercosis:** An infection characterized by cyst-forming tapeworms ingested from infected pork meat.
>
> **Alveolar-Hyatid Disease:** An illness resulting from infection by larvae of the tapeworm species *Echinococcus multilocularis*.

In physical size, tapeworms are the largest of all known intestinal parasites. Tapeworms can survive inside the body for more than 10 years and can grow up to 30 feet in length! Consuming undercooked meat (such as pork, beef, or fish) can pass the parasite on to a human. In the U.S., the beef tapeworm is the most common species to infect people due to the large number of cows infected by eating grasses from contaminated soil or drinking contaminated water.

Did You Know?

Tapeworms in sushi and other raw fish attach to the wall of the intestine and can lay up to 1 million eggs a day! The longest tapeworm ever reported (not certified) was measured at an astounding 37 feet long!

Young parasites penetrate through a cow's intestinal lining and into its bloodstream, eventually making their way into the muscle tissue. The tapeworm then infects the human host after they eat infected meat. Then they attach themselves to the intestinal tract walls to mature and reproduce. Symptoms of tapeworm infection include diarrhea, abdominal cramping, nausea, and severe appetite changes. Unaddressed tapeworm infections in humans can eventually affect other organs and cause diseases such as **Cysticercosis** and **Alveolar-Hyatid Disease.**

DOCTOR'S NOTE:
Regular colon and parasite cleansing can purge tapeworms, their eggs and offspring from your body. See "Parasite Cleansing" in Chapter 12.

Tapeworm Infestation

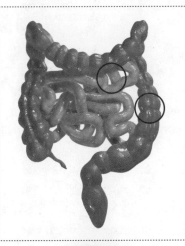

ANATOMICAL OVERVIEW:

Typical sites within the small and large intestines for Tapeworm infestation.

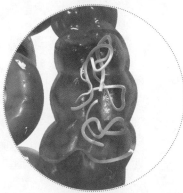

INTERIOR VIEW:

Adult organisms steal important nutrients from the host and reproduce in large numbers.

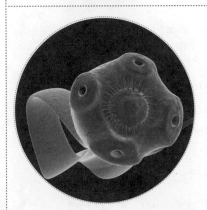

MAGNIFIED VIEW:

A Tapeworm attaches itself to the intestinal lining with microscopic teeth, feeds, and excretes toxic waste matter.

Fig. XX

Roundworm / Pinworm Infestation

ANATOMICAL OVERVIEW:

Typical site within the large intestine for Pinworm infestation. Also, pinworms routinely exit the body via the anal opening.

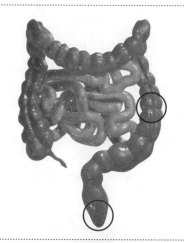

INTERIOR VIEW:

Adult organisms congregate within the host and reproduce in large numbers.

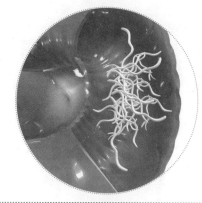

MAGNIFIED VIEW:

Pinworms exit the anus at night to lay their eggs; the host scratches the area and transmits them to the mouth if hands remain soiled.

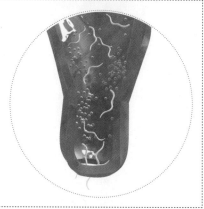

Fig. XXI

Roundworms/Pinworms

Roundworms, sometimes called nematodes, exist as over 20,000 different species. More than 15,000 of these variations are parasitic in nature. **It's estimated over 1.5 billion people are infected with some form of roundworm, making them one of the most common intestinal parasites on the planet.**[123] Hookworms, pinworms, and Trichinella are all types of roundworms that commonly afflict the intestinal tract of humans.

Pinworms *(Enterobius vermicularis)* are small white intestinal parasites believed to specifically target humans. Once inside the body, pinworm eggs are moved along to the small intestine where they hatch and mature. Adult pinworms make their home in the colon where they can live for several months.

Symptoms of a pinworm infection include anal itchiness, insomnia, and poor appetite. Re-infestation can occur continuously (especially in children) because the eggs are laid around the anus and the resulting itchiness causes the host to scratch and then transfer the eggs back to the mouth if hands are not washed thoroughly and often. Transmission is also possible through contaminated clothing, toilets, bed linens, or other surfaces housing these parasites. Pinworm eggs can survive on surfaces outside of the body for up to two weeks and infection occurs if someone touches a contaminated surface, and then places their fingers in the mouth.

With an estimated 40 million people affected, pinworms are the most common intestinal parasite to infect people in the United States.[124] These infections occur all over the world but are seen most frequently in school-aged children living in overpopulated and/or unclean environments.

Hookworms

Hookworms are able to penetrate the human skin. This adaptation allows them to enter the body through the feet of people who walk

Hookworm Infestation

ANATOMICAL OVERVIEW:

Typical sites within the small intestine for Hookworm infestation. Hookworms can enter the body by penetrating the skin of the feet.

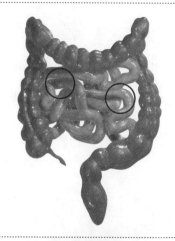

INTERIOR VIEW:

Adult organisms affix to the intestinal lining and can cause illness and conditions such as anemia.

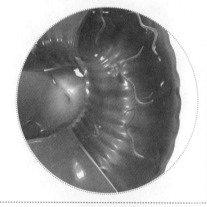

MAGNIFIED VIEW:

A Hookworm attaches itself with razor sharp teeth and begins to ingest blood.

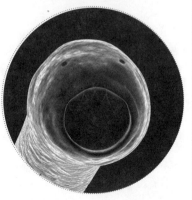

Fig. XXII

barefoot in areas contaminated with fecal matter. Once inside the body, hookworms sink their fangs into the intestinal wall and begin consuming blood. Most infections occur in tropical and subtropical areas where the climate is moist and warm. Symptoms of hookworm infection include stomach pain, loss of appetite, nausea, diarrhea, constipation, bloody stool, gas, itchy skin, fever, and fatigue.

Hookworms can live inside the body for up to 10 years. Prolonged infection can lead to serious symptoms such as iron deficiency (anemia) because the worms excessively suck blood from the intestinal tract. In some cases, the infection can lead to heart problems.

Trichinella

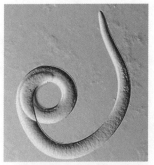

Fig. XXIII: Trichinella viewed under microspcope

The Trichinella worm causes the disease trichinosis and leads to a staggering number of physical ailments such as muscle soreness, fever, diarrhea, nausea, vomiting, edema of the lips and face, difficulty breathing, difficulty speaking, enlarged lymph glands, fatigue, and dehydration. Eating raw or undercooked pork is usually the cause of Trichinella infection in humans. It is most common in areas where pigs are fed raw animal carcasses before being slaughtered for human consumption. In a manner similar to tapeworms, young Trichinella worms encase themselves in the muscle tissue of animals and then mature in a human host once the animal is consumed.

Flukes (Flatworms)

The largest intestinal fluke in humans, *Fasciolopsis buski* makes its home in the upper part of the small intestine. The adult worms produce an average of 25,000 eggs every day. In the past, this fluke was limited to Bangladesh, Cambodia, China, India, Indonesia, Laos, Malaysia, Pakistan, Taiwan, Thailand, and Vietnam. However, with worldwide travel and the importation of contaminated foods and animals, this intestinal fluke is now infecting people worldwide and is spreading rapidly.

Fluke Infestation

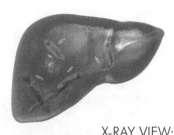
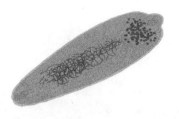

X-RAY VIEW:

Liver flukes *(Clonorchis sinensis)* are trematodes that infest the organ and subsequently cause various negative symptoms.

MAGNIFIED VIEW:

A Liver fluke possesses complex digestive and reproductive systems, with multiple asymmetrical diverticula.

Fig. XXIV

Common symptoms of infestation include abdominal pain, diarrhea, allergies, nausea, vomiting, and intestinal ulcers. Research now suggests this intestinal fluke may even be passed directly from human to human through exchange of bodily fluids during sex, breastfeeding, and other intimate activities.

Liver Flukes exist in many different forms. According to Dr. Hulda Clark's research, the sheep liver fluke *(Fasciola hepatica)* and the human liver fluke *(Clonorchis sinensis)* are the most common cause of infections in humans. Symptoms include general fatigue, intermittent fever, mild jaundice, and pain on the right side of the abdomen below the ribs. (Learn more about Dr. Clark's research by viewing *www.drhuldaclark.org*).

✚ DOCTOR'S NOTE:
After years of clinical experience and research, I firmly believe intestinal and liver flukes contribute significantly to the development of cancer. I also believe these flukes can be found in over 75% of people suffering from degenerative diseases. Why? I have seen dramatic changes in people's health after eliminating these and other harmful parasites from the body. To learn how to cleanse these parasites from the body, read Chapter 12.

How Does Candida Affect My Colon?

Candida albicans is a yeast fungus that naturally inhabits the body. Ninety percent of the fungus can be found in the mouth and intestinal tract. Sometimes, however, Candida can grow out of control and produce devastating effects on the body.

Symptoms of Candida Overgrowth

- Abdominal pain
- Bloating
- Constipation
- Decreased sex drive
- Depression
- Fatigue
- Food allergies
- Hair loss
- Headaches
- Inability to think clearly
- Indigestion
- Itchy eyes
- Menstrual irregularities
- Muscle and joint pain
- Sinus drainage
- Skin rashes
- Toenail and fingernail fungus
- Urinary tract infections
- Weight change

Excessive Candida also robs the body of essential nutrients by consuming starches and sugars in the digestive tract. As Candida consumes food, like any other living organism, it also produces waste. This waste is toxic to the human body and can cause a wide range of symptoms frequently confused with other disorders.

Having a small amount of Candida in your system is not problematic. In fact, a little Candida is a good thing because it acts as a natural antibiotic and helps limit the growth of harmful bacteria. However, using birth control pills or prescription antibiotics (coupled with poor diet patterns, alcohol and soft drink consumption, and general poor health) can easily lead to an overgrowth of this yeast. Drinking chlorinated water can also contribute to Candida's overgrowth because chlorine kills the beneficial bacteria that normally regulate its reproduction. Without enough natural digestive flora in your system, the fungus can proliferate unchecked.

Candida Infestation

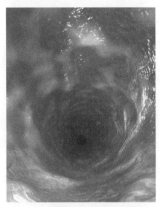

Fig. XXVa: Candida thrives in warm, moist environments and emits toxic waste

➕ DOCTOR'S NOTE:

Because of my extensive research concerning digestive disorders and remedies, I believe Candida overgrowth is rampant. Based on my former private practice and consultation with other health professionals, I estimate 8 out of 10 people have prominent Candida infections that can lead to chronic fatigue and bowel disease if left untreated.

What Bacteria and Viruses are Toxic To My Colon?

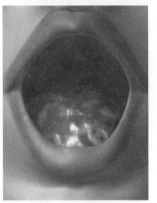

Fig. XXVb: Candida can spread from the intestines into the throat and mouth

The colon naturally accommodates billions of bacteria to help digest starches and convert them into useful fatty acids and other energy products needed for a healthy colon. These good bacteria also help break down nutrients and prevent the growth of harmful bacteria such as the aforementioned Candida.

Certain types of bacteria (such as *Escherichia coli* and *Clostridia*) can putrefy meat within the large intestine, essentially turning it into a cancer-causing agent. This means people who eat large quantities of meat and very little fiber are at an increased risk for developing colon cancer.

E. coli Infestation

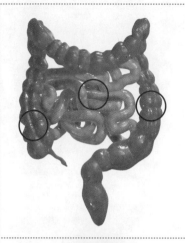

ANATOMICAL OVERVIEW:

Typical sites within the intestinal tract for *Escherichia coli* infestation. The bacteria enter the body when the host ingests water or food contaminated with fecal matter.

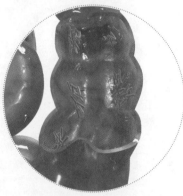

INTERIOR VIEW:

The bacteria inflame and damage the bowel lining which can lead to severe health conditions.

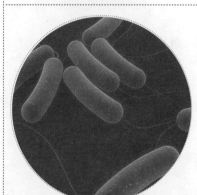

MAGNIFIED VIEW:

A color-enhanced depiction of an E. coli colony as might be viewed under a powerful microscope.

Fig. XXVI

What Happens When E. coli Infects the Colon?

Escherichia coli are a type of bacteria inhabiting the colon. While most strains of E. coli (as it is commonly known) are relatively harmless, others cause serious and sometimes even fatal health problems such as kidney failure and Hemolytic-Uremic Syndrome in children. In Walkerton, Ontario in 2000, E. coli was discovered as the culprit when 160 people sought medical treatment after drinking bacteria in contaminated well water throughout the month of May. By July of the same year, over 2300 people had become ill and at least 6 people had died from ingesting the bacteria. The cause—a farm very close to one of the town's primary water wells had been fertilized with contaminated cow manure and the runoff from heavy rains had easily found its way into the underground water supply. Sadly, the mass outbreak and deaths could have been avoided if simple monitoring procedures already in place had been followed.[125]

E. coli secretes toxins and causes the intestinal tract to become inflamed, which can damage the bowel lining. Undercooked ground beef, and contaminated water, are typical vectors for an E. coli infection. Symptoms of infection include bloody diarrhea, abdominal cramps, nausea, and vomiting.

How Does Clostridium Infect My Colon?

Clostridium difficile is responsible for nearly 3 million cases of diarrhea and colitis (colon inflammation) every year. "Infection with C. difficile is associated with recent use of antimicrobial medications and with residence in hospitals"[126] due to the fact antibiotics can kill necessary digestive flora along with harmful bacteria. C. difficile is transmitted through fecal matter and can survive

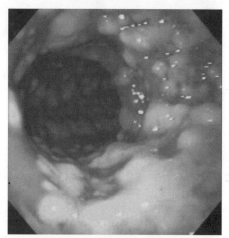

Fig. XXVII: Endoscopic photo view (light enhanced): Example of rampant overgrowth of Clostridium within the human intestinal tract

Salmonella Infestation

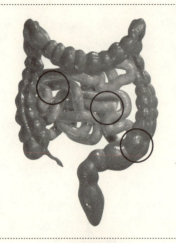

ANATOMICAL OVERVIEW:

Typical sites within the intestinal tract for Salmonella infestation. The bacteria enter the body when the host ingests food or water contaminated with fecal matter.

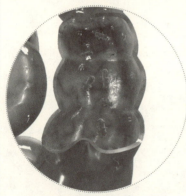

INTERIOR VIEW:

The bacteria cause sickness rapidly with severe negative health symptoms presented.

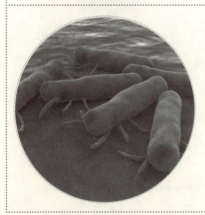

MAGNIFIED VIEW:

Salmonella is a virulent species of bacteria and it can infect multiple organs within the body.

Fig. XXVIII

for up to 70 days outside a host (you). It often contaminates surfaces in hospitals such as bedding and toilets. Severe cases of Clostridium infection can result in septicemia, renal failure, pneumonia, urinary tract infection, and anemia. Frequent foul-smelling stools, abdominal cramps, or bloody stools are also symptoms of a clostridium infection.[127]

What Happens When Salmonella Infects My Colon?

This type of bacteria can cause typhoid fever and intestinal infections in humans (although typhoid is rare in the United States). Salmonellosis is transmitted to humans through consumption of food and water directly contaminated with fecal matter. Therefore, the bacterium can be picked up in a variety of public eateries, not just from preparing raw meat or eggs on your kitchen counter. Once the *Salmonella* bacteria are ingested, symptoms of the infection may become apparent anywhere from 6 to 48 hours later. Symptoms of *Salmonella* infection include headache, diarrhea, abdominal pain, fever, nausea, and vomiting.

In some cases, diarrhea caused by *Salmonella* is so severe the resulting dehydration requires hospitalization. These patients can also develop an inflammation of the intestinal walls. The bacteria can penetrate the walls of the digestive tract, travel via the bloodstream, and then infect other organs of the body. Death is possible from a severe salmonellosis infection but normally occurs only in small children, the elderly, and anyone with a weakened immune system. Around 30,000 cases of culture-confirmed cases are reported to the CDC (Center for Disease Control) every year in the United States. This number may account for about two percent or less of the actual number of infections. The CDC estimates "… 1.4 million cases of salmonellosis occur annually in the United States", making it one of the nation's leading causes of bacterial gastroenteritis.[128]

Warning! These Foods May Contain Salmonella!

- Chocolate

- Coconut
- Fish, shrimp, and frog legs
- Non-pasteurized milk and dairy
- Peanut butter
- Raw meats, poultry, and eggs
- Sauces and salad dressings

Intestinal Toxins from Viruses

If intestinal disease cannot be explained by the organisms listed above, it may be caused by a viral infection. The Rotavirus, Norwalk virus, Cytomegalovirus (CMV), and Sapovirus, among others, can cause gastroenteritis. Viral gastroenteritis (characterized by watery diarrhea) is common worldwide and is easily transmitted by sharing drinks, food, eating utensils, or even toys, bottles, and pacifiers in the case of young children. You can also become ill by eating or drinking a product previously contaminated by a virus.

Food can become contaminated as a result of unsanitary practices (e.g. handling of food products without first washing hands) or from shellfish contaminated with viruses through contact with untreated sewage. Water systems affected by sewage can also pollute public drinking water and, in this manner, viruses can be transmitted to people.

How Do I Avoid These Harmful Organisms?

Your body is subjected to a massive amount of toxins caused by various intestinal invaders every day! Parasites can potentially contribute more toxins to your colon than any other source (food, water, air, etc.). Parasites can live, breed, consume valuable nutrients, and excrete toxic waste inside your body as long as you are alive.

The best defense—a strong and healthy immune system can help repel many of the organisms seeking to invade your body. However, it may be more "proactive" to simply take preventative measures for keeping harmful organisms out of your body in the first place. Study the following tips for avoiding and eliminating parasitic infection—they just may save your life!

How to Reduce Toxins from Parasites

- Wash all fruits and vegetables. Remove any waxy coatings applied to the food's exterior (as a cosmetic preservative). Cut out any "nicked", dark, mushy, or recessed areas in produce. Buy organic foods whenever possible.

- Carefully cook meats, chicken, and fish to the appropriate temperature. Check the food (especially fish) for worms that may be just beneath the skin. Wash hands carefully after handling any raw meat and clean all work surfaces after every food prep. Use a wooden cutting board when preparing or cutting raw meats. Plastic cutting boards do not kill harmful organisms.

- Know your water source. Drink only pure water from a multi-filtered source. Contaminated water is a very common method of infection so it's very important to know the source and quality of the water you drink. Ideally, drink only purified or distilled water supplemented with organic Apple Cider Vinegar for extra nutrients. (See "Apple Cider Vinegar" in the *Resources* section)

How to Reduce Toxins from Parasites (contd.)

- Wash your hands frequently throughout the day. Warm water and natural tea tree soap can help remove any microscopic parasites with which you have come into contact. Clean in and beneath fingernails as well. Especially, wash your hands before and after handling or cooking raw foods, before eating, and after using the toilet, caring for pets, or changing a baby's diaper.

- Keep your living area clean. Parasites can make their home in dust, soil particles, and even the fecal matter from dust mites and cockroaches. Remove dust frequently from surfaces and flooring with a dampened sponge and a HEPA vacuum cleaner respectively. Change your bedding every few days and wash them in hot water. Consider investing in a high quality indoor air filter.

- Wear shoes. Some parasites can penetrate the skin and enter the body through the soles of the feet. Be sure to keep feet covered, especially if you are in an area such as a beach or playground that may contain contaminated animal waste.

- Wear gloves when gardening. Parasites may be lingering in the soil, just waiting for their next host. Wear gloves to avoid direct contact with parasites and wash your hands when finished.

- Be careful where you swim. Never swallow water while you are swimming, whether you are in a river, lake, or public or private swimming pool. Chlorine does not kill many parasites so their presence is entirely possible. Avoid swimming if you have any open cuts or sores.

- Consume a high quality Probiotic on a regular basis to help populate beneficial flora in your digestive system.

- Undergo a thorough parasite cleanse 2 to 3 times a year. The normal life cycle of most parasites is six weeks, so it will take at least that long to complete a thorough cleanse. See Chapter 12 about performing a Harmful Organism Cleanse.

- Practice a balanced diet to regulate your colon pH. (See *Chapter 6–The Colon Diet*)

- Cleanse your colon regularly. A liver/gallbladder flush can also assist in removing toxins associated with parasites and their waste matter.

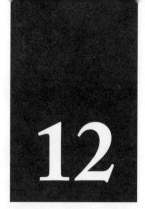

CHAPTER TWELVE

LIVER AND GALLBLADDER CLEANSING, PARASITE CLEANSING, AND HEAVY METAL CLEANSING

As you know by now, the majority of disease is caused by the accumulation of harmful toxins in the body from contaminated foods, beverages, air, water, radiation, prescription medications, negative emotional patterns, and microbes such as bacteria, viruses, worms, mycoplasms, fungus, and yeast.

In this chapter, my goal is to teach you how to heal yourself by activating your own internal self-healing mechanism. The body is the best healing instrument in the world. Our bodies are designed to eliminate any disease!

Disease or poor health typically occurs when your body becomes so contaminated with toxic residue that your internal self-healing mechanism becomes suppressed. To reactivate your self-healing mechanism, you must begin cleansing and purifying your body from years of toxin buildup. You also must follow my recommendations in this book and eliminate the root cause of these toxins from your daily life.

I recommend the following the 4-Step Body Cleanse process to free your entire body of built-up toxic residue.

Dr. Group's 4-Step Body Cleanse

STEP 1
Oxygen Colon Cleanse (6 days)
Start with this cleanse (as outlined in Chapter 5) to clean the entire intestinal tract of years of compacted fecal matter.

STEP 2
Dr. Group's Liver/Gallbladder Cleanse (5 days)
After you have completed the Oxygen Colon Cleanse, perform 3 consecutive Liver and Gallbladder Cleanses (see instructions on the next page). I used to believe 1 liver and gallbladder cleanse was sufficient, but after reviewing thousands of cases, I realized a minimum of 3 and sometimes up to 20 L/G cleanses are required to effectively detoxify the liver and gallbladder and activate the body's self-healing power. In most cases, I wait 5 to 10 days before repeating the Liver and Gallbladder Cleanse, but this depends on the individual and how many toxins they possess. Once you feel up to it, you can begin the 2nd and 3rd cleanse. I also recommend working with a natural healthcare practitioner who can monitor your results and assist you in the healing process.

STEP 3
Dr. Group's Harmful Organism Cleanse (6 weeks)
It's best to start this cleanse after completing the second Liver and Gallbladder Cleanse. This step will take 6 weeks to complete and can be

performed in conjunction with additional Liver/Gallbladder Cleanses and the Heavy Metal Cleanse. **NOTE:** Although I recommend performing this cleanse after the Oxygen Colon Cleanse and 2nd L/G Cleanse, this cleanse can also be performed by itself at any time.

STEP 4
Dr. Group's Heavy Metal Cleanse (6 to 12 months)
After you have completed the third Liver/Gallbladder Cleanse and started on the Harmful Organism Cleanse, I recommend testing yourself with a heavy metal home test kit to see what metals have accumulated in your body. Then, perform the Heavy Metal Cleanse to help flush out mercury, lead, cadmium, aluminum, and other toxic metals.

Before starting the 4-Step Cleansing Process (and so you can monitor your results), I recommend filling out my general **Health Questionnaire** (see *Appendix A*). You may have a long list of symptoms in the beginning but these should slowly begin to disappear after repeated cleansing. I recommend filling out the **Health Questionnaire** again after each L/G Cleanse and after finishing the Harmful Organism Cleanse and Heavy Metal Cleanse to chart your progress.

Dr. Group's Liver/Gallbladder Cleanse

In keeping with my mission to find and develop the best natural and organic products available, I am very pleased to announce I've recently updated my Liver/Gallbladder Cleanse instructions based on the newest and most innovative cleansing formulation, Livatrex™. My extensive research on cleansing herbs has resulted in this organic, ultra-effective liver and gallbladder cleanser.

DOCTOR'S NOTE:
If you do not have a gallbladder, the liver has to work twice as hard and can thus accumulate twice as many stones. This cleanse is highly recommended to help support individuals without gallbladders.

Anatomy of the Liver, Gallbladder, Stomach and Small Intestine

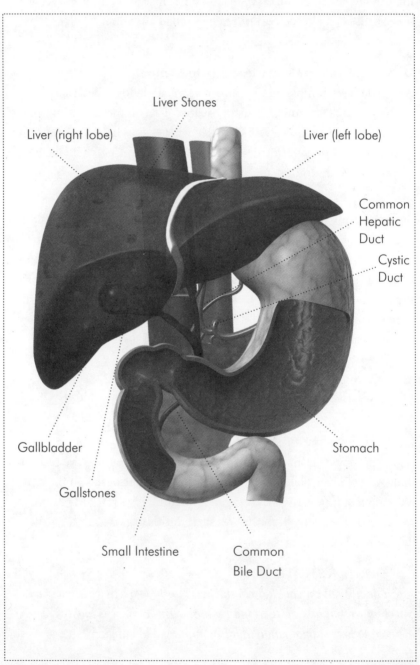

Fig. XXIX

Ingredients for Dr. Group's Liver and Gallbladder Cleanse

- 1 gallon of apple juice (freshly pressed organic). The malic acid in the apple juice helps to soften stones and dissolve stagnant bile that may be present. You can use distilled water instead of apple juice if you are allergic to apples or need to watch your sugar intake due to diabetes

- 2 ounces (1 full bottle) of Livatrex™

- 3 Tablespoons of Epsom salt

- Organic ingredients for making the Liver/Gallbladder Soup

- Organic Fruits for breakfast each morning

- 8 oz. Organic Walnuts or 3 Organic Avocados with 1 Organic Lime or Lemon for the mid-afternoon snack on day 5. (Choose one or the other)

- 6 oz. of Organic Olive oil – Use Extra virgin high quality, cold-pressed for best results

- 1 bottle of Oxy-Powder®

- 1 bottle of Latero-Flora™

- 1 bottle (8 ounces) of Organic Apple Cider Vinegar (available at most health food stores or online)

Instructions: You should be able to perform this liver and gallbladder cleanse while still working or carrying on your normal daily activities. The Oxy-Powder® however can cause watery stools, so make sure a bathroom is nearby. If your stools are liquid, remember this is not diarrhea but the byproduct of turning the solid compacted fecal matter in the intestinal tract into a liquid or gas.

Instructions for Performing the Liver & Gallbladder Cleanse

During the first 4 days of cleansing, I recommend the dietary instructions below or following the "Colon Diet" recommendations in Chapter 6.

1. Eat liver and gallbladder supporting organic fruits for breakfast each morning. These include watermelon, papaya, kiwi, plums, pears, apples, cherries, figs, and grapefruit. For lunch and dinner, eat fresh vegetables, homemade vegetable soups, or salads containing liver and gallbladder detoxifying vegetables such as artichoke, asparagus, carrots, beets, broccoli, cabbage, kale, brussel sprouts, garlic, spinach, romaine lettuce, onions, and cauliflower. Snacks should consist of organic raw seeds or nuts such as sunflower, walnuts, Brazil nuts, or almonds.

2. Avoid drinking coffee, milk, alcohol, bottled juices, or soft drinks during this cleanse. These liquids will decrease the effectiveness of the liver and gallbladder cleanse, and add more toxins to the body. For optimal results drink only distilled water in addition to your cleansing mixture during the day.

It is best to begin the Liver and Gallbladder Cleanse on a Tuesday or Wednesday so on Day 5 (Saturday or Sunday) you will be at home in a relaxing setting and near a bathroom.

DAY 1
MAKE YOUR CLEANSE FORMULA: Add two ounces (the whole bottle) of Livatrex™ and 2 tablespoons of Organic Apple Cider Vinegar to 1 gallon of organic apple juice or distilled water. Shake and refrigerate - You will be drinking this formula for the next 4 days.

During the day drink four 8-ounce glasses of your cleanse formula between meals. **Example:** Drink one 8-ounce glass at 9am, 12pm, 3pm and

6pm. Make sure you drink the mixture 1 hour before or after your meals.

BEFORE BED: Take 4 capsules of Oxy-Powder® and 2 capsules of Latero-Flora™. The Latero-Flora™ will help balance the Probiotic bacteria in the intestinal tract to assist in detoxification.

DAY 2
During the day drink four 8-ounce glasses of your cleanse formula between meals. Make sure you drink the mixture 1 hour before or after your meals.

BEFORE BED: Take 6 capsules of Oxy-Powder® and 3 capsules of Latero-Flora™.

DAY 3
During the day drink four 8-ounce glasses of your cleanse formula between meals. Make sure you drink the mixture 1 hour before or after your meals.

BEFORE BED: Take 6 capsules of Oxy-Powder® and 3 capsules of Latero-Flora™.

DAY 4
During the day drink four 8-ounce glasses of your cleanse formula between meals. Make sure you drink the mixture 1 hour before or after your meals.

BEFORE BED: Take 6 capsules of Oxy-Powder® and 3 capsules of Latero-Flora™.

DAY 5-FLUSH DAY
8 AM to 10 AM: **Breakfast**
Eat a healthy breakfast of organic fresh fruit. Liver supporting fruits include watermelon, papaya, kiwi, plums, cherries, figs, and grapefruit. Choose only one of the fruits above and eat as much as you like between 8 and 10 am. Do not mix the fruits however! If you cannot find fresh fruits, substitute with organic frozen fruit. I recommend using water-

melon if it is available due to its high glutathione content. Start preparing your Liver/Gallbladder Soup for lunch (see the recipe below).

12 PM: Lunch
Choose from one of the following 2 options for your lunch meal.
Lunch Option 1: (Recommended)
To maximize the liver's ability to detoxify and cleanse, I chose a combination of foods which are high in naturally occurring sulphur and glutathione. Sulphur helps the liver detoxify harmful chemicals. The ingredients in the liver gallbladder soup include onions, carrots, garlic, beet, turmeric, and oregano. The combination of these foods will help your liver purge toxins during the cleansing process. Other liver and gallbladder detoxifying foods are artichoke, asparagus, broccoli, cabbage, kale, brussel sprouts, and cauliflower which may also be added to the soup if you wish.

Dr. Group's Organic Liver/Gallbladder Soup

- 1 Organic Beet – Chopped
- 2 Organic Carrots – Chopped
- 10 Organic Garlic Cloves – Minced
- ½ Organic Onion – Chopped
- 1 Teaspoon Organic Himalayan Sea Salt
- ½ Teaspoon Organic Turmeric
- ½ Teaspoon Organic Oregano

Pour 32 ounces of purified water into a soup pot. Add all of the ingredients to the water. Bring to a boil, reduce heat, and then simmer on low heat for one hour. Eat this soup for your lunch meal. After your meal, refrigerate and save the remaining portion of your soup for tomorrow's lunch meal.

Lunch Option 2: (Water Meal)
If you are not hungry or you feel that you can fast through lunch, drink

as much pure distilled water as you can. For every 32 ounces of water you drink during the day add 2 teaspoons of Organic Apple Cider Vinegar.

2 PM: **Mid-Afternoon Snack**
This will be your last meal of the day. Choose one of the following options.

Snack Option 1:
Organic Avocados, Organic Lime or Lemon, and Sea Salt: Eat 3 organic avocados. Season with sea salt and fresh lime or lemon juice to taste. Avocados help the body produce glutathione, which is necessary for the liver to detoxify harmful toxins. Recent studies indicate improved liver health with the regular consumption of avocados.[129]

Snack Option 2:
Eat 8 ounces of raw organic walnuts. Walnuts contain the amino acid arginine, which is necessary to help the liver detoxify ammonia. Walnuts are also high in glutathione and omega-3 fatty acids which support normal liver detoxification. Make sure you chew the nuts well (until they are liquefied) before swallowing.

Snack Option 3:
Water Meal: If you are not hungry or you feel that you can fast through the afternoon, drink as much distilled water as you can. For every 32 ounces of water you drink during the day, add 2 teaspoons of Organic Apple Cider Vinegar.

5 PM: **Epsom Salt**
Mix one and a half level tablespoons of Epsom salt in 8 ounces of warm, purified water. Drink it as fast as you can. It is advisable to be near a bathroom when drinking the Epsom salt as some people experience liquid stools within 20 to 30 minutes after ingestion.

7 PM: **Epsom Salt**
Mix one and a half level tablespoons of Epsom salt in 8 ounces of warm, purified water. Drink it as fast as you can. It is advisable to be near a bathroom when drinking the Epsom salt as some people experience liquid stools within 20 to 30 minutes after ingestion.

9 PM to 10 PM: Olive Oil/Juice

Drink ¾ cup (6 ounces) of organic cold pressed extra virgin olive oil. A small amount (2 tablespoons) of freshly squeezed orange, grapefruit, or lemon juice may be added to improve the taste (optional). Immediately after drinking the oil, go to bed and lie on your right side with your knees drawn up to your stomach for 30 minutes.

After 30 minutes, you can stretch out and go to sleep. If you experience cramping, walk around for ten minutes or so and then go back to bed. You may also feel nauseated during the night. This is due to the release of stored toxins from the gallbladder and liver. This is normal and a sign the Liver and Gallbladder Cleanse is working.

If you feel the need to vomit, do so as this will help release toxins. If you vomit, this is a sure sign your body is extremely toxic and you should consider repeating the Liver and Gallbladder Cleanse after a five day break. Do not take any other supplements on this night.

DAY 6-The Day After the Liver/Gallbladder Flush

Upon waking in the morning, immediately take 4 capsules of Oxy-Powder®. This will help your intestinal tract and body flush the stones released from the liver and gallbladder during the night. For breakfast, eat only fruit. For lunch eat the remaining portion of your liver and Gallbladder Soup. For dinner eat a healthy meal such as a salad and some protein.

Congratulations! You have just completed your first Liver and Gallbladder Cleanse. Stones should appear in your bowel movements for one to two days.

 DOCTORS NOTE:

The best results come with repetition. You will just be scratching the surface of years of accumulated toxins with only 1 Liver and Gallbladder Cleanse. I usually recommend repeating the Liver and Gallbladder Cleanse 3 times

in a row with a break of 5 to 10 days between each session. For someone experiencing a healing crisis (see below), you might want to wait 7 to 10 days between flushes or however long your natural healthcare practitioner recommends.

Repeat the Liver and Gallbladder Cleanse if Necessary.
If you are still experiencing symptoms after your third flush, this may be a sign you need additional cleanses. The most I have heard of someone completing is 20 back-to-back L/G Cleanses before their symptoms were significantly reduced.

Dr. Group's Harmful Organism Cleanse

As stated in Chapter 11, large portions of the population have harmful organisms (parasites) living in their bodies without being aware of it. You can acquire organisms due to many factors such as poor hygiene, consuming unclean produce or undercooked meats, destructive environmental factors, and drinking unsanitary water. Thus, a variety of invaders can be living in your body unknown by you. Such problems can manifest with subtle symptoms that are easily dismissed but can make you quite ill. Changes in skin color, rashes and lesions, changes in bowel habits, an itchy anus, and other signs could be indicative of an invasion by these harmful organisms.

Many people who completed this Harmful Organism Cleanse are amazed at the outcome! You can physically see the result as your waste may begin to include these "unwanted guests" after the cleansing process is initiated. Paratrex® is formulated especially to help flush your system of these harmful organisms. It works by helping to create a hostile environment that is discouraging for these invaders by introducing natural ingredients and organic and wildcrafted herbs into your intestinal system without any harmful effects.

Supplies Needed:
- 2 Bottles of Paratrex®
- 1 Bottle of Latero-Flora™

After completing the Oxygen Colon Cleanse and first Liver/Gallbladder Cleanse, you may begin the Harmful Organism Cleanse. The lifecycle of these harmful organisms, from eggs to full adults, is approximately 6 weeks. For this reason, it is necessary to continue cleansing for the full cycle. The Latero-Flora™ will help create conditions inhospitable to unwanted organisms in the bowel while also promoting a welcoming environment for beneficial intestinal flora that aid in normal digestion.

DAILY FOR 6 WEEKS:
Take 3 capsules of Paratrex® in the morning before breakfast and 3 in the evening before dinner. Take 2 capsules of Latero-Flora™ every other day, first thing in the morning, on an empty stomach, 20 to 30 minutes before breakfast for the entire 6 weeks.

Effective Substances for Parasite Cleansing

 DOCTOR'S NOTE:
I have found that organically certified herbs are twice as potent as standard herbs. They are grown in a clean, toxin-free environment and should be used whenever possible

1. Organic Black Walnut Hull (From Green Hull)
One of the strongest and most versatile herbs for removing parasites, the kernel and green hull are the most potent parts of the Black Walnut to promote parasite cleansing of the intestinal tract. The high tannin content of the green hull is primarily responsible for the walnuts beneficial properties. Other constituents such as juglandin, juglone, and juglandic acid are also involved in the purging process. Some research suggests Black Walnut can oxygenate the blood, which also helps create a hostile environment to parasites. The green husk also contains organic iodine, which possesses antimicrobial properties assisting your intestinal tract in the cleansing of harmful parasites.

2. Organic Male Fern Root
Researchers have determined that male fern root contains the compounds filicin, filmarone, and oleoresin, which help establish an environment toxic to a broad range of parasites in your body.

3. Organic Clove
Clove Bud is considered one of the best herbs for killing parasite eggs and it also acts as a powerful fungicide.

4. Organic Wormwood
References to Wormwood date back to 1600 BC in Egypt. Historically, wormwood has been used as an intestinal cleanser and anti-parasite herb. Wormwood creates an extremely hostile environment for parasites and also promotes healthy digestive processes such as increasing liver and gallbladder secretions.

5. Organic Fresh Water Diatomaceous Earth (DE)
The razor sharp edges of the diatoms in Diatomaceous Earth discourage parasitic colonization of the intestinal tract. These sharp edges slice tiny holes in the parasites' outer shells, causing them to lose vital fluids and die. This natural substance helps the body fight parasites without chemicals. DE won't harm beneficial Probiotic organisms in the bowel, and ingestion of Diatomaceous Earth is not toxic to mammals.

6. Organic Kamala
Kamala has been traditionally used to eliminate intestinal and blood-borne parasites. Kamala is especially useful for eliminating tapeworms and roundworms and is known to act quickly and effectively.

7. Organic Grapefruit Seed Extract
A botanical extract derived from the seeds of wildcrafted or organic grapefruit, the active ingredient (citricidal) of grapefruit seed extract can safely and effectively kill harmful

pathogens. Citricidal can also help create an unwelcoming environment for intestinal invaders.

8. Organic American Wormseed (*Chenopodium*)
Derived from the seeds and other aboveground parts of wormseed, *Chenopodium* is an excellent ingredient for any product used to promote a healthy intestinal environment. Before being popularized by the medical establishment in America during the 19th century, American Wormseed was frequently used by Native Americans to support digestive health. Wormseed is also said to have properties for removing intestinal irritants that cause spasms within the colon wall. Wormseed contains up to 90% ascaridol—an ingredient found to be useful for discouraging parasites.

Other Effective Remedies

Organic Oregano Oil
The subject of numerous academic studies, Oregano Oil contains multiple ingredients that are toxic to harmful microorganisms. For example, a compound found in this healthful oil (carvacrol) provides potent anti-microbial effects, especially for bacteria, and yeast such as *Candida albicans*.

BreviBacillis laterosporus B.O.D. Strain (BBL)
BBL helps maintain a healthy colon and populates the intestines with beneficial bacteria. Latero-Flora™ (a high quality Probiotic containing this strain) has shown incredible effectiveness for easing gastrointestinal symptoms and food sensitivities while also enhancing digestive function. Bacillus is also highly effective for eliminating Candida from the digestive tract.

Bacillus coagulans
Previously known as *Lactobacillus sporogenes*, *Bacillus coagulans* is another very effective Probiotic that helps the body restore the natural balance of micro-organisms in the intestinal tract.

Dr. Group's Heavy Metal Cleanse

As I explained in Chapter 10, every day your body is bombarded with toxins from hazardous metals such as arsenic, aluminum, mercury, lead, cadmium, and more! Dangerous heavy metals and their compounds are stored in body tissue and must be eliminated to help restore the body's self-healing mechanisms. Detoxifying the body is a big step in the right direction, but it must be coupled with an active effort to avoid exposure to heavy metals in the first place.

Before starting the **Heavy Metal Cleanse**, I recommended completing the **Oxygen Colon Cleanse, 3 Liver /Gallbladder Cleanses,** and the first two weeks of the **Harmful Organism Cleanse.** Heavy metal cleansing can take a lot of time so please be patient. It's best to stay on the program for 3 months and then re-test yourself to make sure the levels are being reduced. Removing heavy metals from your system can easily take 6 months to a year or even longer.

STEP 1:
Have yourself tested for heavy metals: Many chiropractors or natural healthcare practitioners can do this for you, either through hair, blood, or urine analysis. You can also order heavy metal (hair and urine) test kits for in-home testing (see "Heavy Metals" in the *Resources* section). I recommend doing this first so you'll have a baseline of your current metal toxicity level. Repeat the test every 3 months to track your progress.

STEP 2:
After extensive research and personal testing of many products, I recommend taking the following products to aid your body in expelling heavy metals and chemical toxins. The products below will allow your body to slowly eliminate these toxins over time.

1. NDF Plus™ (Nanocolloidal Detox Factor Plus)
NDF stands for Nanocolloidal Detox Factors which are designed to help remove toxic metals and harmful substances from the body safely and

effectively. During the process of cleansing, toxins can enter the bloodstream before they exit the body, and this can cause minor health symptoms for people sensitive to the effects of detoxification. As you begin to purge, your body can react with skin blemishes, headaches, general body aches, and other outward signs indicating your body is beginning to rid itself of its chemical burden.

Ingredients of NDF Plus™

Probiotics encourage the growth of beneficial bacteria in the digestive tract, basically by feeding the natural flora in the stomach, colon, and other areas. The natural flora help you break down and digest food and also try to prevent harmful bacteria from propagating in your body.

Organic Milk Thistle helps the liver and the gallbladder flush out harmful toxins, encourages the growth of new cells, and promotes optimal function of these vital organs. Many individuals take Milk Thistle to detox their bodies of residue from alcohol, drugs, and a lifetime of neglectful eating habits. This natural herb also provides antioxidants to help prevent damage of the body's cells by free radicals.

Horsetail has been used topically for thousands of years to treat a variety of minor skin conditions, but it has been discovered to also work as an astringent within the kidney and other organs. Saponins within the plant act upon toxins within the body to help break them down for efficient elimination during the cleansing process.

Himematzutake is a mushroom that has been taken for thousands of years in Asian cultures for promoting a strong immune system. The body's ability to resist disease lies in its physiological fitness and many of Earth's natural resources can help in this regard. Himematzutake works to lower the presence of harmful substances such as fats while encouraging the growth of toxin-destroying cells within the body. Plus, Himematzutake mushrooms provide at least 50 enzymes, 25 vitamins and minerals, and 18 amino acids.

Reishi is a mushroom that can lower blood pressure while assisting the immune system in its task of eliminating harmful toxins from the body. Reishi is also a powerful antioxidant, bactericide, and promoter of normal blood flow. For over 4,000 years, the Japanese and Chinese peoples have consumed Reishi mushrooms to reduce liver dysfunction and support the natural cleansing of toxins from the body.

Cordyceps (also known as *Cordyceps sinensis*) is yet another amazing mushroom shown to improve liver function and help the body resist the effects of free radicals. Cordyceps works by optimizing blood flow to the liver and kidneys, thus enhancing their natural function to better resist the onset of disease.

Fulvic acid is used primarily as a "bioactivator" to enhance the body's natural electrical potential. This allows your internal systems to make better use of natural health supplements by supporting optimal nutrient transmission and assimilation. Fulvic acid has been found to promote electrical activity throughout the body, especially during cell-to-cell communication and within the brain.

Additional Benefits of NDF Plus™

NDF Plus™ is designed to help flush the body of heavy metals and other dangerous toxins; but it does not cause a loss of vital vitamins and minerals. In fact, NDF Plus™ provides multiple nutrients such as amino acids and enzymes. It also helps balance these essential nutrients in the body so you have neither too few nor too many of any given substance.

To summarize, NDF Plus™ provides the following key benefits:
- Helps the body purge heavy metals, pesticides, and other toxic residue
- Contains only organic ingredients such as natural herbs, fungi, and amino acids
- Promotes optimal function of the liver, gallbladder, and other

cleansing organs
- To date, no one has reported ill side effects from taking this supplement
- Can be taken even for extended periods without negative results
- Flushes out harmful chemicals while allowing the body to retain beneficial nutrients
- Supports the growth of natural flora while discouraging the growth of harmful organisms
- Does not cause a toxic overload or "healing crisis" as the toxins are flushed from the organs into the bloodstream for elimination

Dosage: I recommend starting by taking one drop of NDF Plus™ 2 times each day and increasing your dose by one drop every other day until you are taking 15 drops 2 times each day. Continue this dosage for at least 3 to 6 months. You should cease either when that time expires or when most of the toxic metals are fully purged from your body. Take NDF Plus™ on an empty stomach between meals. Also, you should drink plenty of purified water throughout the day whenever cleansing your body of heavy metals.

2. Quantum Zeolite™
Zeolites are a form of volcanic crystal renowned for their ability to absorb toxic materials from aqueous environments. Quantum Zeolite™ is a natural detoxifier formulated from activated zeolite, which is created when molten magma and ocean water fuse together. On the microscopic level, zeolite possesses an infinite number of tiny chambers. When taken internally, zeolites trap toxins within these chambers so they can be easily flushed from the body. Zeolites also retain a wealth of minerals and nutrients from their natural origin (lava and salt water) which you will also benefit from.

Quantum Zeolite™ Contains:
1. Organically concentrated humic acid
2. Natural volcanic zeolite (*clinoptilolite*)
3. Purified water

The Quantum Zeolite™ supplement is superior because it provides zeolites immersed in a highly purified base of organic bio-available humic acid—a complex colloidal molecule used as a chelator to attract and trap harmful metals in the body. Humic acid acts as an internal "detergent" to clean the bloodstream of hydrophobic compounds such as excess salts and lipids. Humic acid also provides organic minerals, such as magnesium and potassium, which are difficult to obtain through diet alone.

Humic acid acts as a transport device to deliver the zeolites everywhere in the body they are needed. After dropping off its zeolite/nutrient payload, the humic acid molecule attaches itself to a heavy metal molecule on the way out, meaning both will be eliminated from the body. The end result is that overall health can be improved with two key functions—providing mineral support for enhanced nutrition and carrying away toxic waste products.

Health Benefits of Zeolites:
- Attracts and absorbs heavy metals and toxins so they can be flushed from the body
- Stimulates the immune system for improved resistance to disease
- Provides essential minerals, vitamins, and other nutrients
- Helps neutralize deadly free radicals (oxidants) within the body
- Supports optimal liver and gallbladder function
- Helps the body absorb energy from food while eliminating waste products
- Balances pH levels, absorbs excess glucose, and neutralizes nitrosamines
- Promotes overall health and wellbeing
- Generally Recognized as Safe (GRAS) by the FDA

Dosage: Take 3 drops 2 times each day or as directed by your healthcare provider. Always dilute the zeolite mixture with a small amount of water (at least 1 teaspoon, not metal) and hold under your tongue for 30 seconds before swallowing. This will facilitate maximum absorption by the body. Take on an empty stomach between meals and drink plenty of purified water throughout the day whenever cleansing your body of heavy metals or toxins.

3. LIFE Detox Foot Patches™

Detox footpads (such as the LIFE Foot Patch™) operate on the principle of withdrawing toxins from the body through the more than 60 acupuncture points found on the soles of your feet. Many natural healthcare practitioners believe toxins travel downward through the body during the day and these special points on the bottom of the foot are directly related to the major organs and systems of the body. LIFE Detox Patches™ takes advantage of this biorhythmic network in a way that is non-invasive yet extremely effective. Furthermore, LIFE Detox Patches™ are manufactured without animal ingredients, harsh chemicals, or other unnatural substances. Combining ancient wisdom with modern technology, LIFE Detox Patches™ are designed to promote the natural detoxification of your body through its own immune system response to foreign matter.

Simply apply LIFE Detox Patches™ to the soles of your feet before going to sleep. LIFE Detox Patches™ work gently while you rest, using the power of proven herbs and natural substances to gently warm and stimulate acupuncture points and meridians. Eastern philosophy teaches these meridians and points covering the exterior of the body, grant access to our internal Chi energy or life force. Once stimulated, these acupuncture points help draw extra energy to various organs and systems that have become weakened through disease and exposure to heavy metals and other toxins.

To explain further, when stimulated properly, your skin's pores can expand to allow the passage of toxic waste out of the body. You can see the visible results of the detoxification by the discoloration of the pads the next morning; they will turn from white to a dark brown or gray tone as they become soiled with toxins. After a while, you may notice the pads being less soiled in the morning, which is a sure sign your body is reducing its toxin load.

Ingredients in the LIFE Detox Foot Patches™

These natural cleansing patches contain no chemical additives, harmful drugs, preservatives, or other artificial substances, but only natural minerals and herbal ingredients such as: Achyranthes Root, Agaricus Mushroom, Balloon Flower, Bamboo Vinegar, Chinese Pea Shrub, Cypress Vinegar, Korean Mugwort, PE+OPP, Siberian Ginseng, Tourmaline, White Peony Root, and Zeolite. The ingredients in LIFE Detox Foot Patches™ work together to help rid the body of accumulated toxins for increased energy, easing of general joint and muscle discomfort, and better rest at night. This unique combination of carefully selected minerals, vinegars, and herbs takes advantage of the body's natural heat emissions (body heat) by reflecting them with a special copper shield back into the foot for improved blood circulation. This exclusive "Heat Reflector" technology thus allows you to more efficiently purge toxins out of your body and into the patches where you want them.

For more information about the health benefits of this product for detoxifying the body, view the entries for "Heavy Metals" in the *Resources* section.

How Do LIFE Detox Patches™ Work?

First of all, LIFE Detox Patches™ are created using only the purest ingredients available and in the proper blending ratios for maximum efficacy. The overall detoxification potential of the ingredients has been optimized by the addition of Tourmaline (a negative ion, far-infrared energy producing mineral) for an unparalleled cleansing experience. The accumulation of heavy metals and chemicals in the body interfere with its ability to absorb essential minerals and vitamins from foods. A lack of proper nutrition can lead to digestive problems, parasitic invasion, occasional to severe allergies, emotional difficulties, chronic illness, and even full diseases.

The Safety Record of LIFE Detox Patches™

In November 2002, The FDA and Texas Department of Health (FSNS) independently certified LIFE Detox Patches™ for application in detecting "non-detectable" heavy metals. Furthermore, LIFE Detox Patches™ do not deliver any drug or chemical into the body; they work topically with natural herbs to stimulate the body's acupuncture points and meridians to encourage the elimination of harmful body toxins. You do not need to take a pill, ingest any mixture, or follow a special diet. However, should you experience any discomfort while using LIFE Detox Patches™, you can simply remove the patches and discontinue use if desired. Feel free to consult with our one of our customer service representatives about your experience or if you have any questions. We have found LIFE Detox Patches™ to be extremely reliable and presenting no ill effects under the recommended guidelines for usage. In fact, LIFE Detox Patches™ can help you in a variety of ways:

Alternative Health Benefits of LIFE Detox Patches™
- Helps you develop more endurance to resist fatigue
- Promotes normal circulation within the body
- Encourages efficient metabolic activity
- Non-invasive—no pill to swallow or mixture to consume
- Economical and convenient—you use them when you decide
- Supports the natural biorhythms of sleep and wakefulness
- Soothes minor body aches by relaxing the area
- Motivates the body's natural release of harmful toxins

Using LIFE Detox Foot Patches™ is a natural way to help your body remove heavy metals, metabolic waste, microscopic organisms, chemical residue, and all kinds of natural and artificial toxins!

Directions:
LIFE Detox Patches™ come with adhesive patches for affixing them to the skin. Although LIFE Detox Patches™ can be safely used anywhere on the body, we recommend applying them to the soles of your feet before going to bed. If your body seems to be carrying an especially heavy toxic load, you can use two pads on each foot until the visible residue has lessened enough that you can rely on just one pad. Be advised—when you check in the mornings, your LIFE Detox Patches™ may be brown, moist,

slightly sticky, and they may emit a foul odor.

Heavy Metals & Toxins Removed by LIFE Detox Foot Patches

- Aluminum
- Antimony
- Arsenic
- Asbestos
- Barium
- Benzene
- Cadmium
- Chlorine
- Cobalt
- Copper
- Fluoride
- Formaldehyde
- Gold
- Isopropyl Alcohol
- Lead
- Mercury
- Methyl Alcohol
- Mold
- Nickel
- Parasites
- PCBs
- Platinum
- Radioactive Materials
- Stainless Steel
- Thallium
- Tin
- Titanium
- Uranium

The results will vary from person to person based on their unique immune system strength, toxic load, and the efficiency of their eliminatory organs. Nonetheless, these are just signs of your body ridding itself of harmful waste and are to be expected. As the pads begin to lighten in color and become less "gooey" after successive use, you will be nearing the end of your detox session. While the cleansing process may take as long as a few months, many people begin noticing positive results and health improvement after just a few days. However, it is advised to continue using the pads now and then to help your body maintain its natural detoxification efforts.

Dr. Group's Closing Statements

So, after everything I have shared with you, I hope you will use this book as a guide for practicing the toxin reduction techniques I provided. Preventing disease and regaining your health begins in the colon. Please share this information with all of your friends, family, and loved ones so they too can learn the secret to health.

If you have any questions, or you would like to speak with one of our award-winning Customer Service Representatives about your health concerns and cleansing programs, you can call our office any time toll-free at 1-800-476-0016.

I wish you the very best in health, and I'm sending you love, peace, happiness, and joy every day!

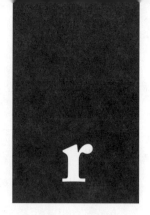

RESOURCES

The following resources are organized alphabetically by major subject heading with product source websites, contact information, and related sub-entries following. We provide healthful alternatives for common foods, personal services, household appliances and materials, and many other organic lifestyle items. Read the corresponding chapter material for each entry to learn more!

Feel free to contact us if you need help finding high quality supplements, you require additional information about any of the following entries, or you have questions about improving your health.

Email: support@ghchealth.com

Telephone: 713-476-0016 or 1 (800) 476-0016

24-Hour Answering Service Available!

Abdominal Massage

Colon Massage (article)
www.colon-cleanse-constipation.com/colon-massage.html

Health-Choices Holistic Massage Therapy School
www.youtube.com/watch?v=3SIhz8W0H-A
1 (908) 359-3995

Maya Abdominal Massage – The Arvigo Techniques™
www.arvigomassage.com
1 (603) 588-2571

Acupuncture

Acupuncture is an alternative healing process involving the insertion of specialized needles just beneath the skin along the body's meridian points. Acupuncturists seek to relieve pain and internal disharmony by stimulating these points to activate or balance the body's *Chi* or life force energy.

Acupuncture
www.acupuncture.com
1 (760) 630-3600

Air Purification

(Air Purification Systems and Filters)

Use a quality air purification system that incorporates UV, negative ions, and HEPA filter technology. Surround Air™ and Way Healthier Home™ are both excellent brands. Also, change your air conditioner filters regularly. I recommend changing the filters every month if you have pets and every other month if you do not.

Online Allergy Relief
www.onlineallergyrelief.com
1 (800) 555-0755

Surround Air™
www.surroundair.com
1 (888) 812-1516

Way Healthier Home™ Air Purifier
www.mercola.com/forms/air_purifiers.htm
1 (877) 985-2695

(Household and Automobile Fresheners)
Use natural air fresheners, not chemical plug-in systems. Beneficial aromatherapy oils include Tea Tree, Citronella, Lavender, Orange and Lemongrass.

Organic and Nature™
www.organicandnature.com

There Must Be A Better Way
www.theremustbeabetterway.co.uk

Alcohol

Detoxify and cleanse your body. Once your body is cleansed, the cravings for alcohol will disappear. Reduce drinking habits to a maximum of one night weekly. The safest alcoholic beverages are unfiltered beer or vodka, but all forms of alcohol are poisons. I highly recommend detoxifying your body of alcohol residue (See Also *Chapter 12—Liver and Gallbladder Cleansing, Parasite Cleansing, Heavy Metal Cleansing*).

Allergies

Seek natural methods for relieving allergies rather than using harmful medications. Note: Organic Oregano Oil is a natural alternative to allergy medications.

NAET® Allergy Elimination Technique
www.naet.com
1 (714) 523-8900

Aloe Vera Juice (Organic)

The structural composition of an Aloe Vera plant includes the very building blocks of life: essential vitamins and minerals, proteins, polysaccharides, enzymes, and amino acids.

Organic Aloe Vera Juice
www.ghchealth.com/aloe_vera_juice.php

R PUR Aloe International® 18X Concentrate
www.rpuraloe.com
1 (800) 888-2563

Antiperspirant (Organic)

Deodorant Stones of America Intl.
www.deodorantstones.com
1 (800) 279-9318

There Must Be a Better Way!
www.theremustbeabetterway.co.uk

Apple Cider Vinegar (Organic)

Apple Cider Vinegar may be one of nature's most potent detoxifiers against a variety of negative health conditions.

Bragg™ Organic Apple Cider Vinegar
www.bragg.com
1 (800) 446-1990

Solana Gold™ Virtues of Vinegar Organic ACV
www.solanagold.com

Spectrum™ Organic Products
www.spectrumorganics.com

Artificial Sweeteners

(See "Sugar" under *Foods*)

Bedding (Organic)

Buy new hypoallergenic bedding every year to prevent the accumulation of droppings, or use organic cotton mattress and pillow casings. (See also "Pillows").

    EcoChoices Natural Living Store
    www.ecobedroom.com
    1 (626) 969-3707

    GREENCulture™
    www.greenculture.com
    1 (877) 204-7336

Biorhythms (Checking Daily Biorhythms)

    Bio-Chart
    www.bio-chart.com

Bristol Stool Scale

The Bristol Stool Scale is a medical tool for classifying bowel movements (as they appear in toilet water) into seven distinct categories. A direct correlation exists between the form of the stool and the amount of time it has spent in the colon (due to factors such as hydration, constipation or lack thereof, diet, etc.).

>Bristol Stool Scale (article)
>www.colon-cleanse-constipation.com/bristol-stool-scale.html

Carpet (Organic Cleaning)

Use non-toxic hardwood flooring or non-toxic wool carpeting. If you cannot afford to replace all your carpet, use all natural carpet cleaning supplies, available at local health-food stores or online.

>Naturell® Carpet and Upholstery Cleaning
>www.bio-techan.com/carpet.htm
>1 (800) 468-3971

>Nirvana Safe Haven
>www.nontoxic.com
>1 (800) 968-9355

>Organic Compounds, Inc.
>www.organiccompounds.com
>1 (800) 448-2933

>Swedry® Carpet Cleaner
>www.swedry.com
>1 (800) 379-2277

>The Vacuum Center.com
>www.thevacuumcenter.com
>1 (877) 224-9998

>These Vacuums Suck
>www.thesevacuumssuck.com
>1 (800) 248-1987

Cellular Devices (and Radiation Protection)

Everyone should have an EMF protection device on his or her cellphone. Learn more about protecting yourself from cellphones with special products.

> Exradia® Wi-Guard
> www.exradia.com
>
> Cellphone Protector
> www.ghchealth.com/cell-phone-emf.php
>
> Mercola Ferrite Beads
> www.mercola.com/forms/ferrite_beads.htm
>
> TOOLS for WELLNESS®
> www.toolsforwellness.com/emf.html
> 1 (800) 456-9887

Chiropractic Resources

Learn about and experience the benefits of chiropractic adjustment and healing methods.

> American Chiropractic Association
> www.amerchiro.org
> 1 (800) 986-4636
>
> International Chiropractic Association
> www.chiropractic.org
> 1 (800) 423-4690

Cleaners and Degreasers (Organic)

> Citrisolve™

www.citrisolve.com
1 (800) 556-6785

GreenEarth® Cleaning
www.greenearthcleaning.com
1 (816) 926-0895

Heather's Naturals & Organic Cleaning Products
www.heathersnaturals.com
1 (877) 527-6601

Seventh Generation™
www.seventhgeneration.com
1 (800) 456-1191

Colon

(General Health, Structure and Function, etc.)

A.D.A.M. Healthcare Center
adam.about.com/encyclopedia/Structure-of-the-colon.htm

The Colon Cleansing and Constipation Resource Center
www.colon-cleanse-constipation.com

(Toxicity and Diseases)

The Colon Cleansing & Constipation Resource Center
www.colon-cleanse-constipation.com
www.colon-cleanse-constipation.com/colon-health

Colon Health Self-Test

A Colon Health Self-Test can be a valuable instrument for providing you with information about the health of your colon as well as your risk of developing serious intestinal problems.

Learn more about your digestive health by taking the test in *Chapter*

Colonic Hydrotherapy

Learn more about colonic hydrotherapy (also known as water colonics).

Colon Hydrotherapy
www.colonic.net
1 (800) 939-1110

International Association for Colon Hydrotherapy
www.i-act.org
1 (210) 366-2888

Cookware (and Avoiding Toxins In)

Avoid aluminum, Teflon®-coated, copper, and cheap stainless steel (inferior grades contain Nickel to reduce costs) cookware. I recommend glass, terracotta (without lead glaze), titanium, silicone, and high quality stainless or cast iron cookware.

Castiron Cookware
www.castironcookware.com

Chef's Resource Silicon Bakeware
www.chefsresource.com

Le Creuset®
www.lecreuset.com/usa/home.php
1 (877) 273-8738

Dust Mites

Check bedding for dust mites in just 10 minutes using the Mite-T-Fast™ home test kit (See Also "Bedding" and "Pillows").

Cleanbedroom.com
www.cleanbedroom.com

Mite-T-Fast™ Allergen Detection System
www.avehobiosciences.com/products.shtml
1 (866) 590-0972

Exercise

I recommend the following exercises and physical activities for helping to reduce stress and improve overall health: Pilates, Qigong (meditative exercise), rebounding, walking, and yoga.

Balanced Body® Pilates
www.pilates.com
1 (800) 745-2837

Cellercise® Rebounding
www.cellercise.com
1 (800) 856-4863

International Association of Yoga Therapists
www.iayt.org
1 (928) 541-0004

Jump 4 Health
www.jump4health.com
1 (888) 815-3332

JumpSport®
www.jumpsport.com
1 (888) 567-5867

National Qigong Association (NQA)
www.nqa.org
1 (888) 815-1893

Qigong Institute

www.qigonginstitute.org

WalkingHealthy.com
www.walkinghealthy.com

Yoga Finder™
www.yogafinder.com
1 (858) 213-7924

Fluorescent Lighting

Replace all fluorescent lighting and standard light bulbs with Full Spectrum or LED lighting.

EcoLEDs
www.ecoleds.com
1 (520) 232-9300

Full Spectrum Solutions
www.fullspectrumsolutions.com
1 (888) 574-7014

Foods (Organic)

Shop at your local farmers' markets. All chain store or national supermarkets stock foods shipped in from distant suppliers. This means the fruit and vegetables are picked before they have ripened and matured to their full nutrient potential. Local farmers' markets, however, pick the food fresh and ripened and deliver it fresh every day or two.

Jaffe Bros. Natural Foods
www.organicfruitsandnuts.com
1 (760) 749-1133

LocalHarvest[sm]
www.localharvest.com

1 (831) 475-8150

Bread (Organic)

Avoid all white, bleached, or enriched breads, pastas, rice, crackers, buns, tortillas, baking crusts, and cereals. Replace these items with whole grains or sprouted grain (wheat) flour. Healthful bread products can be purchased from natural food markets or ordered online.

>Alive and Well
>www.yahwehsaliveandwell.com
>1 (386) 437-0020

>Diamond Organics
>www.diamondorganics.com
>1 (888) 674-2642

>Heartland Mill
>www.heartlandmill.com
>1 (800) 232-8533

Carbonated and Caffeinated Drinks

When you have a craving for sweets or soda, eat fresh fruit such as watermelon or citrus fruits instead. Try mixing equal parts fresh fruit juice and club soda to create your own delicious soft drinks and punches. Replace those beverages with organic coffee substitutes or herbal teas (See Also "Coffee" and "Tea").

Coffee (Organic Replacements)

Substitute store-bought coffee with natural grain coffee—a ground mixture of grains, nuts, dried fruit, and providing only natural flavors—or herbal blends.

>Bambu®
>www.mehndiskinart.com/Bambu_Coffee_Substitute.htm
>1 (250) 664-6483

Caffé Roma™
www.cafferoma.com
1 (415) 296-7662

Pero®
www.internaturalfoods.com/Pero/Pero.html
1 (973) 338-1499

Teeccino®
www.teeccino.com
1 (800) 498-3434

Cooking Oil (Organic)

Replace processed and unhealthful oils with organic sources of virgin coconut oil, olive oil, Grapeseed oil, or almond oil.

Mercola.com Coconut Oil
www.mercola.com/forms/coconut_oil.htm
1 (877) 985-2695

Olio Beato® Demarco Organic Oil
www.organicoil.com/default.aspx
1 (888) 421-6546

Omega Nutrition
www.omeganutrition.com
1 (800) 661-3529

Spectrum® Organics Cooking Oils
www.spectrumorganics.com/?id=6

VeganEssentials
www.veganessentials.com
1-866-888-3426

Wilderness Family Naturals
www.wildernessfamilynaturals.com
1 (866) 936-6457

List of Pesticides (to Avoid in Common Foods and Beverages)

Environmental Working Group
www.ewg.org
1 (510) 444-0973

Meat (Organic Sources)
Always buy organic, range fed, hormone and antibiotic-free meat products.

Applegate Farms
www.applegatefarms.com
1 (866) 587-5858

Blackwing Quality Meats
www.blackwing.com
1 (800) 326-7874

NorthStar Bison
www.northstarbison.com
1 (888) 295-6332

Milk and Dairy (Organic Replacements)
Replace cow's milk with rice milk, fermented soymilk, raw goat's milk, or hemp, almond, cashew, sunflower, or hazelnut milk.

Living Harvest™
www.worldpantry.com/cgi-bin/ncommerce/ExecMacro/livinghar-vest/home.d2w/report
1 (888) 690-3958

Manitoba Harvest™
www.manitobaharvest.com
1 (800) 665-4367

Notmilk
www.notmilk.com
1 (201) 871-5871

Nutiva®
www.nutiva.com/nutrition/recipes/milk.php
1 (800) 993-4367

Organic Pastures™ Fresh Raw & Cultured Dairy & Living Foods
www.organicpastures.com
1 (877) 729-6455

Organic Valley® Farms–Organic Milk, Dairy, Natural Foods
www.organicvalley.coop
1 (888) 444-6455

SwissLand Cheese Co.
www.swisslandcheese.com
1 (260) 589-2761

Why Real Milk?
www.realmilk.com
1 (202) 363-4394

Yaoh Raw Hemp Milk Maker
www.yaoh.co.uk/hemp-milkmaker.html

Natural Food Storage

Store food in non-toxic containers. Use glass Pyrex® containers with silicone lids to reduce contamination from common plastic containers and plastic wraps.

Pyrex®
www.pyrexware.com

Salt

Replace table salt with natural Himalayan Crystal Salt or Celtic Sea Salt.

These organic salt substitutes are natural (not processed by humans).

Himalayan Crystal Salt®
www.himalayancrystalsalt.com
1 (866) 695-1300

Celtic Sea Salt®
www.celticseasalt.com
1 (800) 867-7258

Braggs™ Liquid Aminos
www.bragg.com/products/liquidaminos.html
1 (800) 446-1990

Seafood (Organic Sources)

Consume only seafood from organic sources to avoid possible mercury and other toxic contamination.

Rose Fisheries
www.rosefisheries.com
1 (877) 747-3107

VitalChoice® Wild Seafood & Organics
www.vitalchoice.com
1 (800) 608-4825

Wild Planet Inc.
www.1wildplanet.com
1 (800) 998-9946

Soy (Organic Sources)

Use organic fermented sources such as Natto (fermented soybeans), Tempeh, Tofu, Miso, or Tamari.

Eden® Organic
www.edenfoods.com/store/product_info.php?products_id=107580
1 (888) 424-3336

San-J International, Inc.
www.san-j.com/product_list.asp?id=1
1 (800) 446-5500

SoyBoy®
www.soyboy.com/index.htm
1 (585) 235-8970

Sugar (Organic Replacements)

Replace refined sugars and artificial sweeteners (saccharin, neotame, acesulfame potassium, aspartame, and sucralose) with organic Agave Nectar®, Xylitol®, raw cane sugar, or locally grown unprocessed honey.

Agave Nectar
www.madhavahoney.com
1 (303) 823-5166

Aunt Patty's® Natural Foods & Ingredients
www.auntpattys.com
1 (800) 456-7923

Organic Maple Syrup
www.maplevalleysyrup.com
1 (800) 760-1449

YS Organic Bee Farm
www.ysorganic.com
1 (800) 654-4593

Xylo-Sweet® All Natural Xylitol Sweetener
www.xlear.com/xylosweet
1 (513) 898-1008

For more information on the toxic effects of artificial sweeteners, visit:

Sweet Poison
www.sweetpoison.com

Truth About Splenda
www.truthaboutsplenda.com

Tea (Organic Replacements)

Choice Organic Teas
www.choiceorganicteas.com
1 (206) 525-0051

Numi Organic Tea
www.numitea.com
1 (866) 972-6879

The Republic of Tea®
www.republicoftea.com
1 (800) 298-4832

Water (Organic)

Oxygen water is purified water with the additional benefit of providing oxygen to your system.

hiOsilver Oxygen Water
www.hiosilver.com
1 (650) 493-7874

Fungus/Yeast Remedies

I highly recommend consuming Probiotics (such as *Bacillus laterosporus* and *Bacillus coagulans*) on a regular basis to encourage the growth of beneficial bacteria in the digestive system while also discouraging the growth of harmful organisms. Organic Oregano Oil also works great for fungus and yeast problems!

Fungus Research
www.nail-fungus-toenail.com
1 (512) 706-5657

Latero-Flora™
www.ghchealth.com/probiotic-bacterium-supplement.php
1 (800) 476-0016

Genetically Modified Foods (GMO)

For an extensive list of foods and brands containing GMO's, visit:

The True Food Network
www.truefoodnow.org
1 (415) 826-2770

Geopathic Stress (Natural Solutions)

For clearing geopathic stress, I highly recommend the Safe Space™ 3—a holographic-bar imprinted 20-inch copper tube intended to reduce energy fluctuations to relieve stress. The tube can be buried in the ground near your house to neutralize a 200-acre area of GS.

Protection Solutions
www.safespaceprotection.com/safespace3.htm

Health and Self-Healing

(political activism for)

Alternative Health Insurance Services
www.alternativeinsurance.com
1 (800) 331-2713

Citizens for Health
www.citizens.org
1 (612) 879-7589

Health Freedom Foundation
www.healthfreedom.net
1 (800) 230-2762

Heat Therapy (Far Infrared)

Also known as Far Infrared Therapy (FIR), heat therapy helps dissolve toxins in the blood so you can sweat them out.

Far Infrared Sauna
www.ghchealth.com/health-accessories

TheraSauna™ Dry Infrared Health Sauna
www.therasauna.com
1 (888) 729-7727

Heavy Metals

Heavy Metals (Cleansing Products)

You must cleanse your body of dangerous heavy metals and other harmful toxins to restore or achieve optimal health.

LIFE Detox Foot Patches™
www.ghchealth.com/cleansing
1 (800) 476-0016

NDF Plus™
www.ghchealth.com/cleansing
1 (800) 476-0016

Quantum Zeolite™
www.ghchealth.com/cleansing
1 (800) 476-0016

Heavy Metals (Test Kits)

Receive a hair, saliva, and/or urine analysis to determine if heavy metals are present in your body. We recommend the MineralCheck™ test kit for hair analysis and Osumex for saliva and urine analysis.

> MineralCheck™
> www.ghchealth.com/cleansing
> www.bodybalance.com/mineral/index.asp
> 1 (888) 891-3061
>
> Osumex
> www.ghchealth.com/cleansing
> www.heavymetalstest.com
> 1 (905) 339-2686

Heavy Metals (Vaccine Toxicity)

Take the time to educate yourself, your family, and friends about the dangers of many common vaccines. Learn more about VIC (Vaccine Injured Children) and the dangers of vaccines from Vacinfo.org. Also, study the table "Toxic Ingredients of Common Vaccines" and the related material in *Chapter 9—How to Eliminate Colon Toxins from Drugs and Stress*.

> Autism & Vaccines: A New Look At An Old Story (forum)
> www.ghchealth.com/forum/autism-amp-vaccines-a-new-look-at-an-old-story-discussion-143.php
> 1 (800) 476-0016
>
> BeingHealthyNaturally.com
> www.beinghealthynaturally.com/childrenbabyhealth
> 1 (773) 665-4005
>
> Educate-Yourself
> educate-yourself.org/vcd
> 1 (949) 544-1375
>
> Mothering Mall – Natural Family Living
> www.mothering.com/shop/index.php?target=products&product_id=29791
>
> NewsTarget.com
> www.newstarget.com/vaccines.html

Vacinfo.org
www.vacinfo.org
1 (800) 939-8227

Herbal Medicine Source

American Herbal Products Association
www.ahpa.org
1 (301) 588-1171

Ion Foot Baths (for Detoxification)

A Major Difference
www.ioncleanse.com
1 (877) 315-8638

Ionic Oasis™, LLC
www.ionicoasis.com
1 (402) 806-0699

Microwave Oven (Natural Replacement)

Always grill, steam, broil, or bake your food and replace your microwave with an air-convection oven.

Compact Appliance
www.compactappliance.com
1 (800) 297-6076

Mold and Mildew Control

Use a dehumidifier to help clear moisture out of the air. If you live in a high humidity area, dehumidify the house at least twice a week. In Australia, Tea Tree Oil is commonly used in ventilation systems to control bacteria and mold growth. Also, have your home tested for mold spores, particularly if you live in a humid area.

Use a high quality air purification system that includes UV, negative ions, and HEPA filter technology. The Germicidal UV lamp is the most effective air purification method available for destroying microorganisms like viruses, bacteria, and fungi such as mold (See Also "Air Purification").

IMS Laboratory, LLC.
www.HomeMoldTestKit.com
1 (877) 665-3373

Liberty Natural Products
www.libertynatural.com
1 (800) 289-8427

Mountain Rose Herbs
www.mountainroseherbs.com/aroma/q-z.html
1 (800) 879-3337

Paint (Organic/Non-Toxic)

Purchase non-toxic paints from companies specializing in these products.

Ecos™ Organic Paints
www.ecosorganicpaints.com
Green Planet Paints®
www.greenplanetpaints.com
1 (520) 394-2571

Real Milk Paint®
www.realmilkpaint.com
1 (800) 339-9748

Pesticides and Insecticides (Organic)

Use only natural alternatives to chemical pesticides to avoid putting toxins into your environment.

Arbico Organic
www.arbico-organics.com
1 (800) 827-2847

Beyond Pesticides
www.beyondpesticides.org
1 (202) 543-5450

Pharm Solutions Inc.
www.organicpesticides.com
1 (805) 927-7400

Pets Dander (Removing)

Vacuum and wash all bedding frequently using an all-natural laundry detergent and a vacuum with a HEPA filter. Use an excellent air purification system that includes UV, negative ion, and HEPA filtration (See Also "Air Purification").

Only Natural Pet Store
http://www.onlynaturalpet.com
1 (888) 937-6677

Pet Supplies & Resources (Organic)

Healthy Pet Boutique
ilovemyhealthypet.com
www.healthypetboutique.com
1 (888) 782-8001

The Holistic Pet®
www.theholisticpet.com
1 (888) 452-7263

Pillows (Organic Replacements)

Buy new hypoallergenic pillows every year to prevent the accumulation of droppings, or use organic cotton mattress and pillow casings (See Also "Bedding").

TheCleanBedroom™
www.thecleanbedroom.com
1 (866) 380-5892

NaturalBedStore.com
www.thenaturalbedstore.com
1 (800) 235-3433

Plants

Place living, natural air-cleaning plants in your home. These species include: Boston Ferns, Peace lilies, Arrowhead Vines, Goldon Pothos, English Ivy, Spider Plants, Dracaenas, Areca Palms, and Chrysanthemums.

In the 1980's, NASA experimented with plants by placing them in enclosed rooms containing chemical toxins. Within a 24-hour period, many of the toxins had been digested by the plants and the prior pollution levels were greatly reduced.

The Natural Gardening Company
www.naturalgardening.com/shop/index.php3
1 (707) 766-9303

Organic Plant Care
www.organicplantcare.com
1 (603) 352-8136

Radiation (Detection Devices)

Use a detector such as the (Radalert™ 100) to check the levels of radiation in your home and workplace.

>Radalert™ 100
>www.geigercounters.com/Radalert.htm
>(800) 818-3811

>Tools for Wellness®
>www.toolsforwellness.com
>1 (800) 456-9887

Smoking/Tobacco

You simply MUST quit smoking! You may need a support group to help you so don't give up.

>Foundation for a Smokefree America
>www.anti-smoking.org
>1 (310) 471-4270

>Quitnet® Quit All Together
>www.quitnet.com

>The Stop Smoking Center
>www.stopsmokingcenter.net
>1 (866) 674-2642

Soap (Organic)

To aid in removing microscopic parasites from your skin, wash your hands frequently throughout the day with warm water and natural tea tree soap. Clean in and beneath your fingernails as well.

E3™ Nourishing Soap
www.ghchealth.com/organic-skin-care

Herbaria™ Soap
www.herbariasoap.com

Maggie's Pure Land™ Soap Nuts
www.maggiespureland.com/product.html
1 (888) 762-7688

Soap For Goodness Sake
www.soapforgoodnesssake.com

Squatting Platform (for Proper Bowel Movements)

Lillipad™
lillipad.co.nz

Nature's Platform™
www.naturesplatform.com
1 (828) 297-7561

Swimming Pools (and Chlorine-Free Filtration)

If you have a chlorinated pool, convert it to chlorine free. The ECOsmarte® system uses copper ions and ozone to purify the water. Plus, oxygen naturally detoxifies the body and is also absorbed into the bloodstream for use by the body. Another option is to convert your pool to a saltwater system.

ECOsmarte®
www.ecosmarte.com
1 (800) 466-7946

Toothpaste (Organic)

Find and use healthful alternatives to toxic commercial toothpaste and dental care products. I highly recommend the XyliWhite™ brand—my personal favorite!

> Jason® Natural Toothpaste
> www.jason-natural.com
> 1 (800) 434-4246
>
> Now® XyliWhite™ Toothpaste
> www.nowfoods.com
> 1 (888) 669-3663
>
> Peelu USA
> www.peelu.com
> 1 (800) 457-3358
>
> Philips Sonicare® Toothbrushes
> www.sonicare.com
> 1 (888) 766-4227

Water

Water Filtration

If a whole house water purification unit isn't feasible, install alkalizing and ionizing filters or a full under-sink unit in both the bathroom and kitchen. The Wellness Carafe™ is a high-quality portable water purifier you can take with you anywhere.

> LIFEIonizers™ Alkaline Water for Life
> www.lifeionizers.com
> 1 (888) 688-8889

Wellness Carafe™
www.ghchealth.com/wellness-water-carafe.php

Wellness Kitchen S III Under Sink Conversion Kit
www.ghchealth.com/kitchen-under-sink-conversion-kit.php

Water Testing

You can test your water for contaminants with a home-use water test kit.

PurTest® Kits
purtest.com/2007%20kits.htm
1 (704) 821-3200

Watersafe® Testing Kit
www.ghchealth.com/water-testing-kit.php

ADDITIONAL RESOURCES

Additional Resources

HEALTHCARE PRACTITIONERS

The following alternative and natural medicine practitioners and holistic healers can work with you to determine the causes of your negative health conditions and provide knowledge and/or products to help alleviate them. You may have to perform a little research to see who is in your geographic area.

Block, Keith, M. D.	www.blockmd.com
Briggs, Scott, D.C.	www.mtchirosolutions.com
Brenna, Joseph	www.josephbrenna.com
Brodie, Douglas, M.D.	www.renointegrative.com
Callebout, Etienne, M.D.	(0203) 230 2040
Chopra, Deepak, M.D.	www.chopra.com
Contreras, Ernesto, M.D.	www.oasisofhope.com
Cowden, Lee, M.D.	www.abeim.net
Croft, Don	www.ethericwarriors.com
Day, Lorraine, M.D.	www.drday.com
Diamond, John, M.D.	www.drjohndiamond.com
Donovan, Patrick, N.D.	www.pdonovan.com
Donsbach, Kurt, D.C.	www.hospitalsantamonica.homestead.com
Edelson, Stephen, M.D.	www.edelsoncenter.com
Flanagan, Patrick, Ph.D.	www.phisciences.com
Forsythe, James, M.D.	www.drforsythe.com
Gaby, Alan, M.D.	www.wrightgabynutrition.com
Goldberg, Burton	www.burtongoldberg.com
Group, Jonathan, D.C.	www.austindrx.com
Hoffer, Abram, M.D.	www.islandnet.com/~hoffer
Horowitz, Sir Leonard G., M.D.	www.drlenhorowitz.com
Hudson, Tori, N.D.	www.torihudson.com
Jensen, Bernard, Ph.D.	www.bernardjensen.org
Keller, Helmut, M.D.	www.carnivora.com
Labriola, Dan, N.D.	www.nwnaturalhealth.com

Additional Resources

Lanphier, Loretta, N.D.	www.oasisadvancedwellness.com
Lester, Mark	www.thefinchleyclinic.co.uk
Lipton, Bruce, Ph.D.	www.brucelipton.com
Marcial-Vega, Victor, M.D.	www.marcialvegamd.com
McCabe, Ed	www.oxygenhealth.com
McGraw, Phil, Ph.D.	www.drphil.com
Mercola, Joseph, D.O.	www.mercola.com
Milner, Martin, N.D.	www.cnm-inc.com
Null, Gary, Ph.D.	www.gnhealth.com
Oz, Mehmet, M.D.	www.realage.com
Revici, Emanuel, M.D.	www.revicimedical.com
Rountree, Robert, M.D.	www.boulderwellcare.com
Rubio, Geronimo, M.D.	www.amihealth.com
Schachter, Michael, M.D.	www.mbschachter.com
Simone, Charles, M.D.	www.drsimone.com
Taylor, Jack, D.C.	www.biotor.com
Taylor, Lawrence, M.D.	www.biomedicsinstitute.com
Stoff, Jesse, M.D.	www.drstoff.com
Walker, James R., D.N.H.	1 (334) 514-6950
Weil, Andrew, M.D.	www.drweil.com
Wright, Jonathan, M.D.	www.tahoma-clinic.com

Acupuncture Schools

Note— Information provided by AcupunctureSchools.com, available: www.acupunctureschools.com

Academy for Five Element Acupuncture	Hallandale, FL
Academy of Oriental Medicine at Austin	Austin, TX
Acupuncture & Integrative Medicine College, Berkeley	Berkeley, CA
Acupuncture & Massage College	Miami, FL
American Academy of Acupuncture and Oriental Medicine	Roseville, MN
American College of Acupuncture and Oriental Medicine	Houston, TX
Arizona School of Acupuncture and Oriental Medicine	Tucson, AZ
Dragon Rises College of Oriental Medicine	Gainesville, FL
Eastern School of Acupuncture	Montclair, NJ
Edgewood College of Georgia, School of Oriental Medicine	Norcross, GA
Emperor's College of Traditional Oriental Medicine	Santa Monica, CA
Institute of Clinical Acupuncture and Oriental Medicine	Honolulu, HI
New England School of Acupuncture	Watertown, MA
New York College of Health Professions	Brooklyn, NY
Phoenix Institute of Herbal Medicine & Acupuncture	Phoenix, AZ
RainStar University	Scottsdale, AZ
Southwest Acupuncture College	Albuquerque & Santa Fe, NM
Swedish Institute, College of Health Sciences	New York, NY

Acupuncture Schools

Texas College of Traditional hinese Medicine	Austin, TX
Traditional Chinese Medical College	Kamuela, HI
Tri-State College of Acupuncture	New York, NY
World Medicine Institute, College of Acupuncture and Herbal Medicine	Honolulu, HI
Yo San University of Traditional Chinese Medicine	Los Angeles, CA

Chiropractic Schools

Note—Information provided by ChiropracticSchools.com, available: www.chiropracticschools.com

Cleveland Chiropractic College	Kansas City, MO
Life University, College of Chiropractic	Marietta, GA
National University of Health Sciences	Lombard, IL
New York Chiropractic College	Seneca Falls, NY
Northwestern College	Rancho Cordova, CA
Northwestern Health Sciences University	Bloomington, MN
Palmer College of Chiropractic	San Jose, CA & Port Orange, FL
Parker College of Chiropractic	Dallas, TX
Sherman College of Straight Chiropractic	Spartanburg, SC
Southern California University of Health Sciences, Los Angeles College of Chiropractic	Whittier, CA
Texas Chiropractic College	Pasadena, TX
University of Bridgeport, College of Chiropractic	Bridgeport, CT
Western States Chiropractic College	Portland, OR

Colon Hydrotherapy Schools

Note—All Colon Hydrotherapy schools listed are recognized by the International Association for Colon Hydrotherapy. Information provided by IACT. Available at www.i-act.org/schools.htm

Academy of Colon Hydrotherapy	London, England, UK
Alliance of Classical Teaching	Atlanta, GA
Alder Brooke Healing Arts	Eugene, OR
Angel North England School of Colon Hydrotherapy	Horsforth, UK
Aqua Healing Solutions, Inc.	Hueytown, AL
Aqua Lingua Center for Colon Hydrotherapy Education	Delft, Nederland
Awareness Institute and Natural Wellness Center	Atlanta, GA
Barbara Chivvis Training for Colon Hydrotherapy	Glen Cove, NY
Bekki Medsker School	Quinby, SC
Bethesda Institute	Culver City, CA
Beverly Hills Wellness Center School of Colon Hydrotherapy	Beverly Hills, CA
California Coastal Cleansing Institute	San Diego, CA
Chi Centre Ltd.	Maidenhead, Berks, UK
Chicago School of Colon Hydrotherapy	Chicago, IL
Christian Wellness & Treatment Center	Tyler, TX
Colon Care Hydrotherapy School of Chicago	Chicago, IL
Colonic Copenhagen School of Colon Hydrotherapy	Copenhagen, Denmark

Colon Hydrotherapy Schools (contd.)

Dotolo Institute & ReNew Life School	Tampa, FL
Healing Arts Wellness & Educational Center	Renton, WA
Healing Waters Institute	Burbank, CA
Health Alternatives School of Colon Hydrotherapy	Dayton, OH
Healthymuse School for Holistic Health Practices	Reston/Herndon, VA
Healthy Directions Center	West Hartford, CT
Inner Healings & Assoc, Inc.	Brandon, FL
Internal Environment Institute	Apple Valley, CA
International School of Colon Hydrotherapy, Inc.	Juno Beach, FL
Joyce Long's Wellness Institute	Houston, TX
Las Vegas Colon Hydrotherapy School & Clinic, LLC	Las Vegas, NV
Lifestream Colon Hydrotherapy Institute	Austin, TX
Living In Wellness, LLC	Kihei, Maui, HI
Nevada School of Colon Hydrotherapy	Las Vegas, NV
Nurtura Health Pty Ltd.	Bundaberg, OLD, Australia
Oriental School of Colon Hydrotherapy	Singapore
PPHIC School of Colon Hydrotherapy	North Vancouver, BC, Canada
Saker Clinic / School of Colon Hydrotherapy	Tel-Aviv, Israel
St. John's Academy of Natural Healing & Sciences	Bowie, MD

Colon Hydrotherapy Schools (contd.)

The Art of Health School of Colon Hydrotherapy	Kimberton, PA
The West of England School of Colon Hydrotherapy	Taunton, Somerset, UK
Utah School of Colon Hydrotherapy	Orem, UT
Vestta Whole Health	Vancouver, B.C., Canada
We Care Health Retreat	Desert Hot Springs, CA
Wellness Institute of Colon Hydrotherapy	Denville, NJ

Massage Therapy Schools

Note—Information provided by the Commission on Massage Therapy Accreditation. Available at www.comta.org/sch_directory.html

Academy of Massage Therapy	Hackensack, NJ
Academy of Natural Therapy	Eaton, CO
Academy of Somatic Healing Arts (ASHA)	Norcross, GA
Alexandria School of Scientific Therapeutics	Alexandria, IN
Allegany College of Maryland	Cumberland, MD
American Institute of Massage Therapy	Pompano Beach, FL
Ann Arbor Institute for Massage Therapy	Ann Arbor, MI
Baltimore School of Massage	Linthicum, MD
Blue Cliff College	Baton Rouge, LA
Blue Sky School of Professional Massage	Madison, WI

Massage Therapy Schools

BMSI Institute	Overland Park, KS
Body Therapy Institute	Siler City, NC
Carlson College of Massage Therapy	Anamosa, IA
Cayce/Reilly School of Massotherapy	Virginia Beach, VA
Center for Massage & Natural Health	Weaverville, NC
Cincinnati School of Medical Massage	Cincinnati, OH
Cleveland Institute of Medical Massage	Middleburg Heights, OH
Community College of Rhode Island Therapeutic Massage Program	Newport, RI
Connecticut Center for Massage Therapy	Westport, CT
Cortiva Institute	(Multiple National Locations)
Crystal Mountain School of Therapeutic Massage	Albuquerque, NM
Dayton School of Medical Massage	Dayton, OH
Downeast School of Massage	Waldoboro, ME
East-West College of the Healing Arts	Portland, OR
Educating Hands School of Massage	Miami, FL
Florida College of Natural Health	Miami & Pompano Beach, FL
Florida School of Massage	Gainesville, FL
Healing Hands Institute for Massage Therapy	Westwood, NJ
Health Works Institute	Bozeman, MT
Helma Institute of Massage Therapy	Saddle Brook, NJ
Institute for Therapeutic Massage	(multiple), NJ

Massage Therapy Schools (contd.)

Institute of Therapeutic Massage & Wellness	Davenport, IA
Kishwaukee College, Therapeutic Massage Certification	Malta, IL
Lakeside School of Massage Therapy	Milwaukee, WI
Lakewood School of Therapeutic Massage	Port Huron, MI
Massage Therapy Institute of Colorado	Denver, CO
Mississippi School of Therapeutic Massage	Jackson, MS
Morton College, Therapeutic Massage Program	Cicero, IL
Mountain State School of Massage	Charleston, WV
Mueller College of Holistic Studies	San Diego, CA
The National Massage Therapy Institute	Wilmington, DE
New Hampshire Institute for Therapeutic Arts	Bridgton, ME
Omega Institute – Therapeutic Massage Program	Pennsauken, NJ
Potomac Massage Training Institute	Washington, DC
Roane State Community College – Somatic Therapy Program	Oak Ridge, TN
St. Charles School of Massage Therapy	St. Charles, MO
Sarasota School of Massage Therapy	Sarasota, FL
Solex Medical Academy	Wheeling, IL
Springfield Technical Community College	Springfield, MA

Massage Therapy Schools (contd.)

Synergy Healing Arts Center & Massage School	Blue Ridge Summit, PA
Virginia School of Massage	Charlottesville, VA

Naturopathic Schools

Note—Information provided by NaturopathicSchools.com Available at www.naturopathicschools.com

American Institute of Alternative Medicine	Columbus, OH
Blue Heron Academy	Grand Rapids, MI
California College of Ayurveda	Grass Valley, CA
California Institute for Healing Arts & Sciences	Sacramento, CA
California School of Herbal Studies	Forestville, CA
Complementary and Alternative Medicine Program at Stanford	Stanford, CA
Clayton College of Natural Health	Birmingham, AL
MIND BODY Naturopathic Institute	San Antonio, TX
National College of Naturopathic Medicine	Portland, OR
Pacific College of Oriental Medicine	San Diego, CA
Southwest College of Naturopathic Medicine & Health Sciences	Tempe, AZ
Southwest School for Botanical Medicine	Bisbee, AZ

Naturopathic Schools (contd.)

University of Bridgeport, College of Naturopathic Medicine	Bridgeport, CT
University of California at Berkeley	Berkeley, CA

Additional Natural Health Services, Organizations, and Promoters

The following organizations provide alternative healing strategies, products, and technologies to help you restore or achieve your optimal health. Available: www.i-act.org/schools.htm

Acupuncture.Com	www.accupuncture.com
Alternative Health Insurance Services	www.alternativeinsurance.com
Alternative Health News Online™	www.altmedicine.com
American Academy of Biological Dentistry	www.biologicaldentistry.org
American Association for Health Freedom	www.freedom.net
American Association of Naturopathic Physicians	www.naturopathic.org
American Herbal Products Association	www.ahpa.org
American Holistic Medical Association	www.holisticmedicine.org
Annie Armen Live™	www.anniearmenlive.org
AromaTherapy.com	www.aromatherapy.com
Asset Protection.com (Rob Lambert)	www.assetprotection.com
Bajanor Obesity Center	www.bajanor.com

Additional Natural Health Services, Organizations, and Promoters

Buteyko Breathing Recondition Technique	www.buteykointernational.com
The Cancer Cure Foundation	www.cancure.org
Captured Light Distribution	www.whatthebleep.com
CHIPSA Gerson Medical	www.chipsa.com
Chrisbar Health & Nutrition	www.chrisbar.com
Citizens for Health	www.citizens.org
Clinica IMAQ (Dr. Isai Castillo)	www.drcastillo.com
Cocoon Nutrition Scientific Breakthroughs for Radiant Health (Stephen Heur)	www.cocoonnutrition.org
Conscious Media Network	www.consciousmedianetwork.com
Discount Juicers	www.discountjuicers.com
DMSO.com	www.dmso.com
Dove Clinic for Integrated Medicine	www.doveclinic.com
Drucker Labs Carbon-Bond Organic Nutrition	www.druckerlabs.com
Dynamic Chiropractic	www.dynamicchiropractic.com
Eden Health & Beauty (Emma Bland)	www.eden-healthandbeauty.co.uk
Edgar Cayce Research	www.caycecures.com
Educate-Yourself.org	www.educate-yourself.org
EMC^2 Energetic Matrix Church of Consciousness, LLC.	www.energeticmatrix.com
Environmental Dental Association (Layton, Grant H., D.D.S.)	www.laytondental.com

Additional Natural Health Services, Organizations, and Promoters

Feng Shui Directory of Consultants and Schools™	www.fengshuidirectory.com
Garden Organic	www.gardenorganic.org.uk
Gentle Wind Project	www.gentlewindproject.org
Harold Manner Clinic	www.manner.com.mx
Hay House, Inc.	www.hayhouse.com
The Heart – The Final Destination (Julie Anderson)	www.destinationheart.com
The Heartwork Institute	www.awakentheheart.org
The Hempest	www.hempest.com
Holistic Dental Association	www.holisticdental.org
Homeopathic Educational Services	www.homeopathic.com
Intention Energy Group USA	www.iegroupusa.com
Inversion Table Superstores	www.inversion-table-direct.com
Keep Smiling	www.keepsmiling.com
Kelowna Naturopathic Clinic (Swetlikoff, Lorne, N.D.)	www.natural-medicine.ca
Michael Moore	www.michaelmoore.com
NaturalCures.com (Kevin Trudeau)	www.naturalcures.com
Natural Awakenings Healthy Living	www.naturalawakeningsmag.com
Natural Fibers	www.natural-fibers.com
The Norwalk Juicer	www.norwalkjuicer.com
Oprah Winfrey	www.oprah.com
Organic Consumers Association	www.organicconsumers.org
Organic Trade Associatio	www.ota.com

Additional Natural Health Services, Organizations, and Promoters

OxyHealth	www.oxyhealth.co.uk
Poly-MVA® Palladium Lipoic Complex™ (Garnett, Merrill, M.D.)	www.polymva.com
Price Chiropractic & Nutrition Center (Price, Patrick, D.C.)	www.drpatrickprice.com
QualityHealth	www.qualityhealth.com
Quantum-Touch	www.quantumtouch.com
The Raw Food World	www.therawfoodworld.com
Raw Guru	www.rawguru.com
The Rolf Institute of Structural Integration	www.rolf.org
ROM – The 4-Minute CrossTrainer©	www.fastexercise.com
Saunders-Matthey Cancer Prevention Coalition	www.stopcancer.org
Sonic Bloom For The World	www.sonicbloom.com
Stella Maris Clinic	www.stellamarisclinic.com
Stem Enhance	www.stemenhance.com
StopCancer.com (Wayne Graham)	www.stopcancer.com
SunGazing.com	www.sungazing.com
Suzanne Somers	www.suzannesomers.com
Tetrahedron Publishing Group (Horowitz, Leonard G., M.D.)	www.tetrahedron.org
The Meatrix	www.themeatrix.com
Trader Joe's	www.traderjoes.com

Additional Natural Health Services, Organizations, and Promoters

USDA Organic Program	www.ams.usda.gov/nop/indexNet.htm
Webspirit New Age Spiritual Growth EBooks	www.webspirit.com
Westfall Foundation	www.westfallfoundation.org
Weston A. Prince Foundation	www.westonprince.org
Whole Foods® Market	www.wholefoodsmarket.com
Yerba Prima Dry Skin Brushes	www.yerbaprima.com
YS Organic Bee Farm	www.ysorganic.com

Watch the DVD of The Secret and/or read the book!
This valuable information can help you change your outlook and approach to mastering life by giving you the "secret" to manifesting all your dreams and goals! The following teachers are featured in The Secret and I highly recommend reading their books, adopting their philosophies, and following their methods for improving the quality of your life!

John Assaraf, Michael Beckwith, Lee Brower, Jack Canfield, John F. Demartini, Marie Diamond, Mike Dooley, Bob Doyle, Hale Dwoskin, Morris E. Goodman, John Gray, John Hagelin, Bill Harris, Ben Johnson, Loral Langemeier, Lisa Nichols, Bob Proctor, James Arthur Ray, David Schirmer, Marci Shimoff, Joe Vitale, Denis Waitley, Neale Donald Walsch, and Fred Alan Wolf.

Available:
As DVD – www.ghchealth.com/thesecretdvd
As Book – www.ghchealth.com/thesecretbook

Recommended Reading

Author	Title
Angell, Marcia, M.D.	The Truth About Drug Companies: How They Deceive Us and What to Do About It
Balch, Phyllis A., C.N.C	Prescription for Nutritional Healing – Fourth Edition
Batmanghelidj, E., M.D	Water Cures: Drugs Kill: How Water Cured Incurable Diseases
Bechamp, Antoine	The Blood and its Third Anatomical Element (1912)
Becker, Robert, M.D. and Gary Selden	The Body Electric – Electromagnetism and the Foundation of Life
Bell, Fred, Ph.D.	Rays of Truth – Crystals of Light
Brennan, Barbara Ann,	Hands of Light – A Guide to Healing Through the Human Energy Field
Bryson, Christopher	The Flouride Deception
Ciaramicoli, Arthur, Ph.D. and Katherine Ketcham	The Power of Empathy
Covey, Stephen R.	The 7 Habits of Highly Effective People
Daniel, Kaayla T., Ph.D.	The Whole Soy Story
Day, Lorraine	AIDS--What the Government Isn't Telling You

Recommended Reading

Author	Title
Diamond, John, M.D. and W. Lee Cowden, M.D.	An Alternative Medicine Definitive Guide to Cancer
Emoto, Massaro	Messages from Water
Fitzgerald, Randall	The Hundred-Year Lie – How Food and Medicine are Destroying Your Health
Fried, Stephen	Bitter Pills: Inside the Hazardous World of Legal Drugs
Gordon, Richard	Quantum-Touch – The Power to Heal
Gustafson, Eric	The Ringing Sound – An Introduction to the Sound Current
Haley, Danie	Politics in Healing
Hay, Louise L.	You Can Heal Your Life
Horowitz, Sir Leonard G., M.D.	Healing Codes of the Biological Apocalypse
Jampolsky, Gerald, M.D. and Diane Cirincione	Change Your Mind, Change Your Life
Jarvis, DeForest Clinton, M.D.	Folk Medicine
Johnson, Julian	The Path of the Masters
Karp, Reba Ann	Edgar Cayce Encyclopedia of Healing

Recommended Reading

Author	Title
Kelley, William D., D.D.S.	One Answer to Cancer with Cancer Cure Suppressed
Lewis, Stephen & Evan Slawson	Sanctuary – The Path to Consciousness
Moss, Ralph W., Ph.D.	The Cancer Industry
Myss, Caroline, Ph.D.	Anatomy of the Spirit
Orloff, Judith, M.D.	Dr. Judith Orloff's Guide to Intuitive Healing
Quillin, Patrick, Ph.D.	Beating Cancer with Nutrition
Robbins, Anthony	Unlimited Power: The New Science of Personal Achievement
Talbot, Michael	The Holographic Universe
Tracy, Brian	Time Power
Truman, Karol K.	Feelings Buried Alive Never Die …
Walker, James R., D.N.H.	Holocaust American Style
Work, Rich (with Ann Marie Groth)	Awaken to the Healer Within

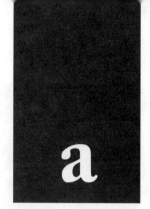

APPENDIX **A**
HEALTH QUESTIONNAIRE

Use this Questionnaire to gauge your progress before and after cleansing.

Fill this out right before you start cleansing and every 60 days while cleansing

INSTRUCTIONS:

1. Circle YES or NO to answer the questions.
2. Fill in Your Score where indicated.
3. Save this questionnaire to compare your results from before and after cleansing.

General Health Questionnaire

Today's Date: _____

Overall Well-Being

Consider Your Current Symptoms and Overall Sense of Well-Being and Answer:

Do You Feel Healthy?   Yes   No

Do You Consider Yourself Happy?   Yes   No

List any negative health symptoms you're experiencing:

_____

_____

_____

Do You Have Chronic Inflammation in Your Body?

If You Answer 3 or More Questions "YES" You May Have Chronic Inflammation.

Do you have elevated cholesterol or triglycerides?   Yes   No

Do you have numbness or tingling in your arms or legs?   Yes   No

Do you eat meat, commercially baked sweets, fried foods, or use vegetable oil daily?	Yes	No
Do you consume fish less than two times per week?	Yes	No
Do you have high blood pressure, asthma, or colitis?	Yes	No
Do you smoke?	Yes	No
Do you have gingivitis or periodontal disease, or not have regular dental cleansings and check-ups at least once every six months?	Yes	No

What is your score?
Add up the number of "YES" and "NO" responses: _____

Poor Nutrition and Lifestyle

Do You Have Poor Nutrition and Digestion?
If You Answer 4 or More Questions "YES" You May Have Poor Nutrition and Digestion.

Do you regularly include fast food in your diet (three or more times per week)?	Yes	No
Do you experience belching, bloating, or persistent fullness soon after eating, or do you experience excess gas often?	Yes	No
Do you experience heartburn or acid reflux two or more times per week?	Yes	No
Are you allergic to any specific foods?	Yes	No
Do you feel fatigued or lethargic after eating?	Yes	No
Do you commonly have bad breath or a bad taste in your mouth?	Yes	No

Do you use digestive aids such as laxatives, antacids, or acid-blocking drugs?   Yes   No

Do you often feel "older" than you should for your age?   Yes   No

Does your skin look sallow, gray, puffy, wrinkled, or aged?   Yes   No

> **What is your score?**
> **Add up the number of "YES" and "NO" responses:** _____

Do You Have Abnormal Blood Sugar Levels? Are You Pre-Diabetic or At Risk?

If You Answer 3 or More Questions "YES" You Could Have Abnormal Blood Sugar Levels.

Does your waistline extend beyond your hips or are you overweight?   Yes   No

Do you become tired or light-headed or do you feel the need to eat again just two or three hours after your last meal?   Yes   No

Do you eat dried beans e.g. pinto, navy, black, etc. less than three times per week?   Yes   No

Do you exercise less than three times each week?   Yes   No

Do you eat two or more servings of bread, pasta, candy, colas, or fruit juice a day?   Yes   No

Do you eat fewer than five servings of fresh, raw vegetables and fruits per day?   Yes   No

Do you have high blood triglyceride levels or suffer from hypertension?   Yes   No

> **What is your score?**
> Add up the number of "YES" and "NO" responses: _____

Do You Have Impaired Cellular/Mitochondrial Function?

If You Answer 3 or More Questions "YES" You May Have Impaired Cellular Function.

Are you frequently tired for no reason (especially around 3 PM)?	Yes	No
Do you have stiff and/or sore muscles (unrelated to recent exercise)?	Yes	No
Do you have poor stamina, shortness of breath, or feel exhausted after exercising?	Yes	No
Do you exercise less than two hours per week?	Yes	No
Have you ever been diagnosed with iron deficiency or do you have heavy menses (for women)?	Yes	No
Do you look older than your true age?	Yes	No
Have you ever been exposed to toxic chemicals or heavy metals?	Yes	No

> **What is your score?**
> Add up the number of "YES" and "NO" responses: _____

Exposure to Toxins

Is Your Detoxification Capacity Impaired?
If You Answer 4 or More Questions "YES" Your Body Needs Help to Detoxify.

Do you become physically ill when exposed to strong smells (perfume, auto-exhaust, cigarette smoke, etc.)?	Yes	No
Do you use chemical cleaners or solvents at home, at work, or in your hobbies?	Yes	No
Do you live in a house/apartment or work in an office less than 5 years old?	Yes	No
Do you have any amalgam (mercury) dental fillings?	Yes	No
Are you prone to side effects from medications or supplements, or have you become more sensitive to the effects of alcohol or caffeine (reduced tolerance)?	Yes	No
Do you have fewer than 2 bowel movements daily?	Yes	No
Do you smoke?	Yes	No
Do you have or have you ever had breast implants?	Yes	No
Do you have any pets, especially dogs, cats, birds, or other furred or feathered animals?	Yes	No
Do you wake up often during the night to urinate?	Yes	No

What is your score?
Add up the number of "YES" and "NO" responses: ____

Is Your Home and/or Work Environment Toxic?

If You Answer 4 or More Questions "YES" Your Home or Office Needs a "Health Makeover."

Do you have carpet in your home?	Yes	No
Do you vacuum less than 3 times per week?	Yes	No
Have you changed or cleaned your air filters in the		

last 30 days?	Yes	No
Do you routinely drink tap water?	Yes	No
Are your clothes and bedding washed in unfiltered city water?	Yes	No
Have you recently repainted your home on the inside?	Yes	No
Have you noticed any black spots or mold on your air vents or walls?	Yes	No
Do you clean your air vents fewer than 2 times a year?	Yes	No
Do you use chemical based cleaners in your home?	Yes	No
Do you use chemical fertilizers, insecticides, or pesticides?	Yes	No
If your home does not contain a quality air purification system, circle Yes.	Yes	No

What is your score?
Add up the number of "YES" and "NO" responses: _____

Impaired Immune System

What is the Quality of Your Immune System Function?
If You Answer 4 or More Questions "YES" Your Immune System May be Overworked.

Do you catch colds or the flu easily?	Yes	No
Do colds, flu, or other infections tend to linger in your system more than 5 days?	Yes	No
Do you have a chronic cough, scratchy throat, sinus congestion, or excess mucous production making it		

necessary to clear your throat often?	Yes	No
Do you have seasonal allergies or known allergies to dust, animals, or mold?	Yes	No
Have you ever been diagnosed with an autoimmune disease?	Yes	No
Do you have dark circles under your eyes?	Yes	No
Do you have difficulty seeing at night, or do you have white spots on your fingernails?	Yes	No
Have you recently had any vaccinations, including flu shots?	Yes	No
Have you or anyone in your family served in the military in the last 15 to 20 years?	Yes	No

What is your score?
Add up the number of "YES" and "NO" responses: _____

Is Your Liver Impaired by Your Emotions?

If You Answer 5 or More Questions "YES" Your Liver May Be Impaired.

Do you feel angry from time to time?	Yes	No
Are you agitated easily?	Yes	No
Do you have frequent mood swings?	Yes	No
Is it hard to stay in a good mood?	Yes	No
Do you run out of energy during the day?	Yes	No
Do you have brown spots on your skin or age spots?	Yes	No

Does your skin break out or is it blemished?	Yes	No
Are your emotions often on a "roller coaster"?	Yes	No
Do you later have to apologize for your bad moods to friends, family, co-workers, etc.?	Yes	No
Is there always "something wrong" in your life?	Yes	No
Have you ever been physically or sexually abused?	Yes	No
If you are upset, is it best not to talk to you about what's going on?	Yes	No
Do you get annoyed by the "fake" cheeriness of others?	Yes	No
Do these questions irritate you?	Yes	No

What is your score?
Add up the number of "YES" and "NO" responses: _____

Are Your Kidney and Urinary Systems Functioning Properly?

If You Answer 5 or More Questions "YES" Your Kidneys May Be Overworked.

Do you have pain in your muscles and joints?	Yes	No
Have you had kidney or bladder infections in the last year?	Yes	No
Have you experienced ankle pain or swelling in the last year?	Yes	No
Do you have left shoulder pain?	Yes	No
Do your fingernails chip or break easily?	Yes	No

Do you have puffiness, "bags", or dark circles under your eyes?	Yes	No
Is your hair thinning?	Yes	No
Do you have frequent scalp irritations?	Yes	No
Do you have painful, harsh menstrual cycles?	Yes	No
Do you wake up often during the night to urinate?	Yes	No
Do you feel exhausted in the morning even after sleeping 8 or more hours?	Yes	No
Have you ever been diagnosed with thyroid problems?	Yes	No

What is your score?
Add up the number of "YES" and "NO" responses: _____

Do You Have Parasites, Viruses, Fungi, or other Microbes Inside Your Body?

If You Answer 4 or More Questions "YES" You May Need a Thorough Harmful Organism Cleanse.

Do you have any yellowish discoloration on your fingernails or toenails?	Yes	No
Do you have athlete's foot or noticeable foot odor?	Yes	No
Do you have a history of yeast infections?	Yes	No
Have you been "mouthed", scratched, or licked by an animal in the last 6 months?	Yes	No
Have you been bitten by mosquitoes or bugs?	Yes	No
Do you feel bloated, grumpy, or gassy after meals?	Yes	No

Have you eaten at a sushi bar, salad bar, or buffet recently?	Yes	No
Have you ever picked food up off the floor and eaten it?	Yes	No
Do you often crave sugar, sweets, or bread?	Yes	No
Do you experience anal itching?	Yes	No
Do you have dandruff?	Yes	No
Do you have indoor pets?	Yes	No

What is your score?
Add up the number of "YES" and "NO" responses: ____

Hormonal Imbalance

Are Your Adrenal Glands Functioning Properly?
If You Answer 3 or More Questions "YES" Your Adrenal System May Be Suffering.

Do you frequently feel "stressed out"?	Yes	No
Do you have difficulty falling asleep or maintaining sleep through the night?	Yes	No
Do sudden noises make you jump?	Yes	No
Do you become dizzy or light-headed when standing up too quickly?	Yes	No
Do you crave salt or sugar?	Yes	No
Do you drink coffee?	Yes	No
Have you taken any diet pills in the last 3 years?	Yes	No
Do you drink any highly caffeinated beverages such		

as soft drinks or energy drinks?	Yes	No
Do you exercise less than 3 times per week?	Yes	No

> **What is your score?**
> Add up the number of "YES" and "NO" responses: ____

Is Your Thyroid Imbalanced?

If You Answer 4 or More Questions "YES" Your Thyroid May Be Imbalanced.

Are you frequently cold or do you have cold hands and feet?	Yes	No
Do you have trouble "getting going" in the morning?	Yes	No
Do you often feel sad or depressed, especially in the morning?	Yes	No
Are you unable to lose weight despite improving your diet and exercising more?	Yes	No
Do you have "patches" of hair loss on your head, arms, or legs?	Yes	No

> **What is your score?**
> Add up the number of "YES" and "NO" responses: ____

Are Your Sex Hormones Reduced in Production or Quality?

If You Answer 2 or More Questions "YES" Your Sex Hormones May Be Reduced.

Are you "flabby" or have you experienced a loss of muscle tone?	Yes	No
Do you suffer from a low sex drive?	Yes	No
Do you frequently experience headaches or migraines?	Yes	No
Do you have Pre-Menstrual Syndrome (PMS)?	Yes	No

What is your score?
Add up the number of "YES" and "NO" responses: _____

FOR WOMEN—Is Your Body Out of Balance?

If You Answer 6 or More Questions "YES" Your Body is Out of Balance!

Are you very easily fatigued?	Yes	No
Do you suffer from Pre-Menstrual Syndrome (PMS)?	Yes	No
Do you have painful menses (periods)?	Yes	No
Do you frequently experience depression before or during menstruation?	Yes	No
Is your menstrual cycle prolonged in duration or excessive in terms of blood flow?	Yes	No
Are your breasts overly sensitive or "painful" before, during, or after menses?	Yes	No
Do you menstruate too frequently (more than once per month or sporadic flow)?	Yes	No
Do you produce a vaginal discharge?	Yes	No
Have you had a hysterectomy or had your ovaries removed?	Yes	No

Do you have menopausal "hot flashes"?	Yes	No
Is your menses irregular or absent altogether?	Yes	No
Do you have acne or other skin blemishes that worsen during menses?	Yes	No
Have you felt depressed for 3 months or longer?	Yes	No
Do you have hair growth on your face or body?	Yes	No
Do you have or desire sex less than 2 times each month?	Yes	No

> **What is your score?**
> **Add up the number of "YES" and "NO" responses:** _____

FOR MEN—Is Your Body Out of Balance?

If You Answered 6 or More Questions "YES" Your Body May Be Out of Balance!

Are you very easily fatigued?	Yes	No
Do you have premature ejaculation?	Yes	No
Is urination difficult or do you "dribble" i.e. can't stop completely?	Yes	No
Have you experienced or are you experiencing prostate trouble?	Yes	No
Do you often wake up during the night to urinate?	Yes	No
Do you have pain on the inside of your legs or heels?	Yes	No
Do you have feelings of incomplete bowel evacuation or "not emptying fully"?	Yes	No

Do you have problems sleeping?	Yes	No
Do you avoid even routine or mild physical activity?	Yes	No
Do you run out of energy during the day?	Yes	No
Do you experience leg nervousness or "twitching" at night?	Yes	No
Do you have difficulty falling asleep or maintaining sleep through the night?	Yes	No
Have you felt depressed for 3 months or longer?	Yes	No
Do you have or desire sex less than 2 times each month?	Yes	No

What is your score?
Add up the number of "YES" and "NO" responses: _____

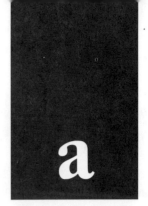

APPENDIX B
ILLUSTRATIONS

PART ONE

Figure I. Healthy Colon, Global Healing Center, Inc. © 2007, pg 3.

Figure II. Appendix. Global Healing Center, Inc. © 2007, pg 5.

Figure III. Anatomy of the Colon. Global Healing Center, Inc. © 2007, pg. 16.

Figure IV. Leaky Gut Syndrome. Global Healing Center, Inc. © 2007, pg. 19.

Figure V. Comparison of Healthy and Unhealthy Colons. Global Healing Center, Inc. © 2007, pg. 21.

Figure VI. Diverticula. Global Healing Center, Inc. © 2007, pg. 35.

Figure VII. Ulcerative Colitis Viewed During Colonoscopy. Released to Public domain, pg. 41.

Figure VIII. Colon Polyp Viewed During Colonoscopy. pg. 43.

Figure IX. Colon Cancer. Global Healing Center, Inc. © 2007, pg. 45.

Figure X. The Bristol Stool Chart. Global Healing Center, Inc. © 2007, pg. 51.

Figure XI. Oxygen Colon Cleanser Breaking Down Toxic Buildup. Global Healing Center, Inc. © 2007, pg. 69.

Figure XI. Benefits of Oxygen in the Body. Global Healing Center, Inc. © 2007, pg. 70.

Figure XIII. Enema Bag Kit. Used with permission of http://www.EnemaKit.com, all rights reserved, pg. 97.

Figure XIV. Colon Hydrotherapy Room. Used with permission of International School for Colon Hydrotherapy, Inc., All rights reserved, pg. 100.

Figure XV. Lillipad™. Used with permission of http://lillipad.co.nz., all rights reserved, pg. 104.

Figure XVI. Mini-Trampoline by ReboundAIR™. Used with permission of ReboundAIR., all rights reserved, pg. 105.

Figure XVII. Organic Goji Borries. Image licensed from IStock.com, Global Healing Center, Inc. © 2007, all rights reserved, pg. 121.

PART TWO

Figure I. Milk...Is It Really So Good?, Global Healing Center, Inc. © 2007, pg 139.

Figure II. Himalayan Sea Salt. Image licensed from IStock.com, Global Healing Center, Inc. © 2007, all rights reserved, pg. 151.

Figure III. Empure Sugar Inc. Global Healing Center, Inc. © 2007, pg. 163.

Figure IV. Smog trapped over Los Angeles. Image licensed from IStock.com, Global Healing Center, Inc. © 2007, all rights reserved, pg. 180.

Figure V. Electron microscopic view of mold spore colony. Global Healing Center, Inc. © 2007, pg. 188.

Figure VI. Pet Dander in Carpet. Global Healing Center, Inc. © 2007, pg. 191.

Figure VII. Magnified View of a Dust Mite. Used with permission of Glen Needham PH.D, The Ohio State University, all rights reserved, pg. 193.

Figure VIII. Benefits of Water in the Body. Global Healing Center, Inc. © 2007, pg. 199.

Figure IX. 2001. United States Geological Survey-Arsenic concentration in U.S. Homes. Used with permission of U.S. Geological Survey 2007, all rights reserved, pg. 202.

Figure X. Counterthink Cartoon. Used with permission of www.newstarget.com, all rights reserved, pg. 204.

Figure XI. Vaccines- The Hidden Poison. Global Healing Center, Inc. © 2007, pg. 221.

Figure XII. The Pressures of Modern Education. Global Healing Center, Inc. © 2007, pg. 226.

Figure XIII. Mercury Dental Filling Vapors. Used with permission of David Kennedy DDS, all rights reserved, pg. 241.

Figure XIV. Cellphones Transmit Intense Radiation. Used with permission of BIOPRO Technology, all rights reserved, pg. 250.

Figure XV. The Modern Skyline of Disease. Global Healing Center, Inc. © 2007, pg. 252.

Figure XVI. Consecutive Stages of Parasitic Infestation. Global Healing Center, Inc. © 2007, pg. 264.

Figure XVII. Giardia Infestation. Global Healing Center, Inc. © 2007, pg. 267.

Figure XVIII. Toxoplasma Infestation. Global Healing Center, Inc. © 2007, pg. 269.

Figure XIX. Cyclospora Infestation. Global Healing Center, Inc. © 2007, pg. 270.

Figure XX. Tapeworm Infestation. Global Healing Center, Inc. © 2007, pg. 272.

Figure XXI. Roundworm/Pinworm Infestation. Global Healing Center, Inc. © 2007, pg. 273.

Figure XXII. Hookworm Infestation. Global Healing Center, Inc. © 2007, pg. 275.

Figure XXIII. Trichinella. Used with permission of Christian Gautier of Vernafilm, all rights reserved, pg. 276.

FigureXXIV. Fluke Infestation. Global Healing Center, Inc. © 2007, pg. 277.

Figure XXV. Candida Infestation. Global Healing Center, Inc. © 2007, pg. 279.

Figure XXVI. E. Coli Infestation. Global Healing Center, Inc. © 2007, pg. 280

Figure XXVII. Example of Rampant Overgrowth of Clostridium within the Human Intestinal Tract. Used with permission of Gregory Ginsberg MD., all rights reserved, pg. 281.

Figure XXVIII. Salmonella Infestation. Global Healing Center, Inc. © 2007, pg. 282.

Figure XXIX. Anatomy of the Liver, Gallbladder and Small Intestines. Global Healing Center, Inc. © 2007, pg. 292.

Special thanks to:

Sebastian Kaulitzki of Carbon Lotus. www.sciepro.com for original medical illustrations.

Jason Salvaggio, www.jasonsalvaggio.com, for cartoons.

BIBLIOGRAPHY

PART ONE

1 California HealthCare Foundation. "Snapshot Healthcare Costs 101." Vol. 4 (2-4). Pub. 2007. Online. Accessed: 9 July 2007. Available as PDF: www.chcf.org/documents/insurance/HealthCareCosts07.pdf

2 Addiss, David G., Shaffer, N., Fowler, Barbara S., and Robert V. Tauxe. "The Epidemiology of Appendicitis and Appendectomy in the United States." American Journal of Epidemiology. Vol. 132, Issue 5. (910-25). Pub. 1990.

3 Arhan P., Devroede G., Jehannin B., Lanza M., Faverdin C., Dornic C., Persoz B., Tétreault L., Perey B., and D. Pellerin. "Segmental colonic transit time." Diseases of the Colon and Rectum. Vol. 24, Issue 8. (625-9). Pub. Nov/Dec. 1981. Online. Accessed: 10 July 2007. Available: www.ncbi.nlm.nih.gov/sites/entrez?cmd=search&db=pub med (PMID=7318630).

4   Rao, S. S. C., "Constipation: Evaluation and Treatment." <u>Gastroenterology clinics of North America</u>. Vol. 32, Issue 2. (659-83). Jun 2003. Available: www.gastro.theclinics.com/article/PIIS0889855303000268/fulltext

5   Adams P.F., Hendershot G.E., and M. A. Marano. "Current estimates from the National Health Interview Survey, 1996." National Center for Health Statistics. <u>Vital H Statistics</u>. Vol. 10, Issue 200. Pub. 1999.

6   Consumer Healthcare Products Association. "OTC Sales by Category—2003-2006." Updated April 2007. Online. Accessed 10 July 2007. Available: www.chpa-info.org/ChpaPortal/PressRoom/Statistics/OTCSalesbyCategory.htm

7   National Cancer Institute. "US Estimated Complete Prevalence (Including Counts) on 1/1/2004." Updated Nov 2006. Online. Accessed 7 Nov 2007. Available: www.srab.cancer.gov/prevalence/canques.html

8   Rona, Zoltan P. "Altered Immunity & Leaky Gut Syndrome." American Fitness Professional & Associates. Pub. 17 Nov 2006. Accessed 7 Nov 2007. Available: www.afpafitness.com/articles/altered-immunity-leaky-gut-syndrome/85

9   National Center for Health Statistics. "Prevalence of Overweight and Obesity Among Adults: United States, 2003-2004." Online. Accessed 11 July 2007. Available: www.cdc.gov/nchs/products/pubs/pubd/hestats/overweight/overwght_adult_03.htm

10   Ibid.

11   Teflon® is a registered trademark of E. I. du Pont de Nemours and Company.

12   Hungin, A. P. S., Chang, L., Locke, G. R., Dennis, E. H., and V. Barghout. "Irritable Bowel Syndrome in the United States: Prevalence, Symptom Patterns and Impact." <u>Alimentary Pharmacology & Therapeutics</u>. Vol. 21, Issue 11. (1365-75). Pub. 2005. Online. Accessed 12 July 2007. Available: www.medscape.com/viewarticle/506173

13 Baker, Danial E. "Rationale for using serotonergic agents to treat irritable bowel syndrome." <u>American Journal of Health-System Pharmacy.</u> Vol. 62, Issue 7. (700-11). Pub. Apr 2005. Online. Accessed 7 Nov 2007. Available for Purchase: www.ajhp.org/cgi/content/full/62/7/700

14 Jones, R. and S. Lydeard. "Irritable bowel syndrome in a general population-Tips from Other Journals." <u>American Family Physician</u>. Vol. 304. (87). Pub. 1992. Online. Accessed 12 July 2007. Available: www.findarticles.com/p/articles/mi_m3225/is_n6_v45/ai_12308986

15 Ibid.

16 Salzman, H. and D. Lillie. "Diverticular Disease: diagnosis and treatment." <u>American Family Physician.</u> Vol. 72. (1229-34). Pub. 2005. Online. Accessed 12 July 2007. Available: www.findarticles.com/p/articles/mi_m3225/is_7_72/ai_n15798326

17 Burt C. and S. Schappert. "Ambulatory care visits to physician offices, hospital outpatient departments, and emergency departments: United States, 1999–2000." National Center for Health Statistics. <u>Vital Health Statistics.</u> Vol. 13. (157). Pub. 2004.

18 Salzman, H. and D. Lillie. "Diverticular Disease: Diagnosis and Treatment."

19 Fasano, A., et al. "Prevalence of Celiac Disease in At-Risk and Not-At-Risk Groups in the United States–A Large Multicenter Study." <u>Archives of Internal Medicine.</u> Vol. 163, Issue 3. Pub. 10 Feb 2003. Online. Accessed 7 November 2007. Available: www.archinte.ama-assn.org/cgi/content/full/163/3/286

20 University of Chicago Celiac Disease Program. "Fact Sheets about Celiac Disease." (From: Fasano et. al., <u>Archives of Internal Medicine</u>. February 2003). Updated March 2005. Online. Accessed 12 July 2007. Available as PDF: www.uchicagokidshospital.org/pdf/uch_007937.pdf

21 Ibid.

22 Loftus, E. "Clinical Epidemiology of Inflammatory Bowel Disease: Incidence, Prevalence, and Environmental Influences." Vol. 126, Issue 6. (1504-17). Pub. May 2004. Online. Accessed: 12 July 2007. Available: www.gastrojournal.org/article/PIIS0016508504004627/fulltext

23 Crohn's & Colitis Foundation of American. "Fact Sheet – Surgery for Crohn's Disease." Updated 2006. Online. Accessed 12 July 2007. Available: http://www.ccfa.org/info/surgery/surgerycd

24 Nachimuthu, S., Piccione, P., and P. Balasundaram. "Crohn Disease." Online. Accessed 13 July 2007. Available: www.emedicinehealth.com/crohn_disease/article_em.htm

25 MayoClinic.com "Ulcerative colitis." Pub. 17 Aug 2007. Online. Accessed 7 Nov 2007. Available: www.mayoclinic.com/health/ulcerative-colitis/DS00598/DSECTION=4

26 National Cancer Institute. "A Snapshot of Colorectal Cancer." Updated Sept 2006. Online. Accessed 13 July 2007. Available as PDF: www.planning.cancer.gov/disease/Colorectal-Snapshot.pdf

27 National Cancer Institute. "Estimated New Cancer Cases and Deaths for 2007." Online. Accessed 13 July 2007. Available as PDF: www.seer.cancer.gov/csr/1975_2004/results_single/sect_01_table.01.pdf

28 Ibid.

29 Ibid.

30 Ibid.

31 Lewis, S. J. and K. W. Heaton. "Stool form scale as a useful guide to intestinal transit time." <u>Scandinavian journal of gastroenterology.</u> Vol. 32, Issue 9. (920-4). Pub. 1997.

32 Colon Cleanse and Constipation Resource Center. "Bristol Stool Scale." Online. Accessed 16 July 2007. Available: www.colon-cleanse-constipation.com/bristol-stool-scale.html

33 Adams, P., Hendershot, G., and M. Marano. "Current estimates from the National Health Interview Survey, 1996."

34 Bannerjee, A., Majowicz, S., Hall, G., Jones, T., Daly, L., Kirk, M. and F. Angulo. "Prevalence of Diarrhea in the Community in Australia, Canada, Ireland and the United States." Online. Accessed 21 Aug 2007. Available as PDF: www.cdc.gov/foodborne/publications/240-scallan_2004.pdf

35 Edgar Cayce. "Reading 1703-2." Online. Accessed 16 July 2007. Available: www.are-cayce.com/th/tharchiv/therapies/colonic.html

36 Solana Gold™ is a registered trademark of Solana Gold Organics. Available: www.solanagold.com

37 Bragg™ is a registered trademark of Bragg Live Food Products, Inc. Available: www.bragg.com

38 Spectrum™ is a registered trademark of Spectrum Organic Products, Inc. Available: www.spectrumorganics.com/

39 At this time, it is unknown whom owns the registration for Homozon.

40 Oxy-Powder® is a registered trademark of Global Healing Center, LP. Available: www.oxypowder.com

41 Oxypowder.com "Germanium-132-Studies." Pub. May 2007. Online. Accessed 8 Nov 2007. Available: www.oxypowder.com/germanium-132-studies.html

42 Todar, K. "The Composition of Normal Flora." Todar's Online Textbook of Bacteriology. Pub. 2002. Online. Accessed 8 Nov 2007. Available: www.textbookofbacteriology.net/normalflora.html

43 Pelka, R., Jaenicke, C. and J. Gruenwald. "Impulse Magnetic-field Therapy for Migraine and Other Headaches: a Double-Blind, Placebo-Controlled Study." Advances in Therapy. Vol. 18, Issue 3. (101-9). Pub. May/June 2001. Online. Accessed 8 Nov 2007. Avail-

able: www.ncbi.nlm.nih.gov/sites/entrez?cmd=search&db=pubmed (PMID=11697020)

44 Consumer Healthcare Products Association. "OTC Sales by Category—2003-2006."

45 Duphalac® is a registered trademark of Solvay S.A. Available: www.www.duphalac.com

46 Kristalose® is a registered trademark of Cumberland Pharmaceuticals, Inc. Available: www.kristalose.com

47 Actilax® is a registered trademark of Alphapharm Available: www.alphapharm.com.au

48 Sorbilax® is a registered trademark of Pharmacia Corp. (purchased by Pfizer Canada Inc. in 2003) Available: www.pfizer.ca/english/home/highres/default.asp?s=1

49 MiraLAX® is a registered trademark of Schering-Plough HealthCare Products, Inc. Available: www.miralax.com/default.html

50 Phillip's® is a registered trademark of Bayer Corp. Available: www.bayercare.com/htm/philhome.htm

51 Dulcolax® is a registered trademark of Boehringer Ingelheim Heathcare. Available: www.dulcolaxusa.com/us/Homepage.jsp

52 Freelax® is a registered trademark of Wyeth Consumer Healthcare Available: www.freelaxrelief.com

53 Fleet® is a registered trademark of C.B. Fleet Company, Inc. Available: www.cbfleet.com

54 Rite Aid® is a registered trademark of Rite Aid Corp. Available: www.riteaid.com/

55 Traditional Medicinals® is a registered trademark of Traditional Medicinals. Available: www.traditionalmedicinals.com/

56 ex-lax® is a registered trademark of Novartis Consumer Health, Inc.

Available: www.ex-lax.com

57. Senokot® is a registered trademark of Purdue Products, L.P. Available: www.senokot.com/html/main/index.asp

58. Nature's Way® is a registered trademark of Nature's Way Products, Inc. Available: www.naturesway.com/NaturesWay/default.aspx

59. Swan® Castor Oil is a registered trademark of Cumberland-Swan, Inc. Available: www.cumberlandswan.com

60. Now Foods® is a registered trademark of NOW® Foods. Available: www.nowfoods.com

61. Correctol® is a registered trademark of Schering Plough Health Care Products, Inc. Available: www.correctol.com

62. Fleet Bisacodyl® is a registered trademark of CB Fleet Co. Available: www.cbfleet.com

63. Dulcolax® is a registered trademark of Boehringer Ingelheim Consumer Healthcare. Available: www.dulcolaxusa.com/us/Homepage.jsp

64. Gentlax® is a registered trademark of Purdue Pharma. Available: www.purdue.ca/main

65. RiteAid® Corrective Laxative Tablet is a registered trademark of Rite Aid Corporation. Available: www.riteaid.com/pharmacy/monographs/drug_search.jsf

66. Metamucil® is a registered trademark of Procter & Gamble. Available: www.metamucil.com

67. Benefiber® is a registered trademark of Novartis AG, Basel, Switzerland. Available: www.benefiber.com

68. Citrucel® is a registered trademark of GlaxoSmithKline. Available: www.citrucel.com

69. The Colon Cleansing & Constipation Resource Center. "Psyllium

Research." Pub. Feb 2007. Online. Accessed 8 Nov 2007. Available: www.colon-cleanse-constipation.com/psyllium-research.html

70 The Colon Cleansing & Constipation Resource Center. "Senna Research." Pub. Feb 2007. Online. Accessed 8 Nov 2007. Available: www.colon-cleanse-constipation.com/senna-research.html

71 Ibid.

72 The Colon Cleansing & Constipation Resource Center. "Cascara Sagrada Research." Pub. Feb 2007. Online. Accessed 8 Nov 2007. Available: www.colon-cleanse-constipation.com/cascara-sagrada-research.html

73 Ibid.

74 Qing-Yi, Lu, et al. "Inhibition of prostate cancer cell growth by an avocado extract: role of lipid-soluble bioactive substances." The Journal of Nutritional Biochemistry. Vol. 16, Issue 1. (23-30). Pub. Jan 2005. Online. Accessed 8 Nov 2007. Available for Purchase: www.sciencedirect.com/science/journal/09552863

75 Bragg™ is a registered trademark of Bragg Live Food Products, Inc. Available: www.bragg.com

PART TWO

1. Picard, Andre. "Today's fruits, vegetables lack yesterday's nutrition." Public Health Reporter. Pub. 6 July 2002. Online. Accessed: 24 July 2007. Available: www.andrepicard.com/whatyoueat.html

2. Ibid.

3. Ibid.

4. James, C. "Global Status of Commercialized Biotech/GM Crops: 2006." ISAAA Briefs. Vol. 35. Pub. 2006. Online. Accessed 6 Nov 2007. Available for Purchase: www.isaaa.org/resources/publications/briefs/35

5. Wertheim, M. "Pharm Phresh: Frankenfoods II." LA Weekly. Pub. Oct 2002. Online. Accessed: 25 July, 2007. Available: www.lawweekly.com/general/quark-soup/pharm-phresh/10271

6. Drucker, Steven M. (Juris Doctor). "Why Fda Policy on Genetically Engineered Foods Violates Sound Science and U.S. Law." Statement delivered at the FDA Public Meeting, Washington, D.C. 30 Nov. 1999. Online. Accessed 30 July 2007. Available: http://www.biointegrity.org/fdaPMP.html

7. Pusztai, A. "Genetically Modified Foods: Are They a Risk to Human/Animal Health?" Online. Accessed 30 July 2007. Available: www.actionbioscience.org/biotech/pusztai.html

8. Gold, Mary V. (Compiler). "Organic Production/Organic Food: Information Access Tools." USDA Definition and Regulations. Pub. June 2007. Online. Accessed 30 July 2007. Available: www.nal.usda.gov/afsic/pubs/ofp/ofp.shtml

9. United States Environmental Protection Agency. "America's Children and the Environment: A First View of Available Measures." Document # EPA 240-R-00-006. Pub. Dec 2000. Pp. (32-3). Online. Accessed 30 July 2007. Available as PDF: www.yosemite.epa.gov/ochp/ochpweb.nsf/content/ACE-Report.htm/$file/ACE-Report.pdf

10 Ibid.

11 Ibid.

12 Ibid.

13 Curl, C., Fenske, R. and K. Elgethun. "Organophosphorus Pesticide Exposure of Urban and Suburban Preschool Children with Organic and Conventional Diets." <u>Environmental Health Perspectives</u>. Vol. 111, Issue 3. Pub. Mar 2003. Online. Accessed 8 Nov 2007. Available as PDF: www.ehponline.org/members/2003/5754/5754.pdf

14 Eskenazi, B., Bradman, A. and R. Castorina. "Exposures of Children to Organophosphate Pesticides and Their Potential Adverse Health Effects." <u>Environmental Health Perspectives</u>. Vol. 107, Issue S3. Pub. June 1999. Online. Accessed 8 Nov 2007. Available for Purchase: www.ehponline.org/docs/1999/suppl-3/toc.html

15 The Codex Alimentarius Commission. "Code of Ethics for International Trade in Food." (Preamble) Rev. Jan 1985. Online. Accessed 30 July 2007. Available as PDF: www.codexalimentarius.net/download/standards/1/CXP_020e.pdf

16 The World Trade Organization at Cancún. "Agriculture and the Environment." Online. Accessed 30 July 2007. Available: www.sierraclub.ca/national/programs/sustainable-economy/trade-environment/wto-cancun-agriculture-env.html

17 Cyocel® is a registered trademark of OHP, Inc. Available: www.ohp.com/Products/cycocel.php

18 Cohen, R. "Eating Blood and Guts-Feeding Dead Cows to Animals." Online. Accessed 30 July 2007. Available: www.notmilk.com/forum/530.html

19 English, D., MacInnis, R., Hodge, A., Hopper, J., Haydon, A., and Graham Giles. "Red Meat, Chicken, and Fish Consumption and Risk of Colorectal Cancer." <u>Cancer Epidemiol Biomarkers</u>. Pub. Sept. 2004. Vol. 13, Issue 9. (1509-14). Online. Accessed 30 July 2007.

Available as PDF: www.cebp.aacrjournals.org/cgi/reprint/13/9/ 1509

20 Animal Place. "Cattle: Not so free on the range." Online. Accessed 31 July 2007. Available: www.animalplace.org/cattle.html

21 Ibid.

22 Animal Place. "Factory Farming: What does it mean?" Online. Accessed 31 July 2007. Available: www.animalplace.org/factoryfarm.html

23 Epstien, S. "Potential public health hazards of biosynthetic milk hormones." International journal of health services : planning, administration, evaluation. Vol. 20, Issue 1. (73-84). Online. Accessed 8 Nov 2007. Available: www.ncbi.nlm.nih.gov/sites/entrez?cmd=search&db=pubmed (PMID=2407676)

24 Ibid.

25 Ibid.

26 Chao, A. et al. "Meat Consumption and Risk of Colorectal Cancer." JAMA. Vol. 293, Issue 2. (172-82). Pub. Jan 2005. Online. Accessed 8 Nov 2007. Available as PDF: www.jama.ama-assn.org/cgi/reprint/293/2/172.pdf

27 Anonymous. "The Dark Side Of Recycling." Pub. in Earth Island Journal. Online. Accessed 3 Aug 2007. Available: www.preciouspets.org/rendering.htm

28 Dr. Joseph Mercola. "Newest Research On Why You Should Avoid Soy." Online. Accessed 6 Aug 2007. Available: www.mercola.com/article/soy/avoid_soy.htm

29 Michael F. Jacobson, Ph.D. "Press Conference on Salt: the Forgotten Killer." Pub. 24 Feb 2005. Online. Accessed 6 Aug 2007. Available as PDF: www.cspinet.org/new/pdf/final_mj_salt_statement.pdf

30 Sasaki, S., Zhang, Xin-Hua and Hugo Kesteloot. "Dietary Sodium, Potassium, Saturated Fat, Alcohol, and Stroke Mortality." Stroke.

Pub. 1995. Vol. 26. (783-9).

31 Truthinlabeling.org "Where is MSG hidden?" Online. Accessed 7 Aug 2007. Available: www.truthinlabeling.org/II.WhereIsMSG.html

32 Charles de Coti-Marsh. "Prescription for Energy." Pub. 1990. Pp. 48. Online. Accessed 7 Aug 2007. www..arthriticassociation.org.uk/pages/home_treatment/downloads/Charles_de_Coti-Marsh_-_Prescription_for_Energy.pdf

33 Kaufman, Marc. "WHO to Talk About Food Carcinogen Finding." *The Washington Post*. Pub. 27 Apr 2002. Online. Accessed 7 Aug 2007. Available: (Contact *Washington Post* Archives).

34 Wayne, A. and L. Newell. "Radiation Ovens-The Proven Dangers of Microwaves." Orig. pub. by *The Christian Law Institute*. Online. Accessed 7 Aug 2007. Available: www.curezone.com/foods/microwave_oven_risk.asp

35 Teflon® is a registered trademark of E. I. du Pont de Nemours and Company. Available: www.teflon.com/NASApp/Teflon/TeflonPageServlet?pageId=/consumer/na/home_page.jsp

36 Michael F. Jacobson, Ph.D. "Liquid Candy–How Soft Drinks are Harming Americans' Health." Pub. 2005 by the Center for Science in the Public Interest. Pp. 8-9. Online. Accessed 8 Aug 2007. Available as PDF: www.cspinet.org/new/pdf/liquid_candy_final_w_new_supplement.pdf

37 Ibid.

38 Ibid.

39 American Beverage Association. "Beverage Industry Basics." Online. Accessed 8 Aug 2007. Available: www.ameribev.org/about-aba/beverage-industry-basics/index.aspx

40 Marylou Doehrman. "Marketing company brings business partners

to schools." <u>Colorado Springs Business Journal</u>. Pub. 14 Nov. 2003. Online. Accessed 8 Aug. 2007. Available: www.findarticles.com/p/articles/mi_qn4190/is_20031114/ai_n10044767. Coca-Cola® is a registered trademark of The Coca-Cola Company.

41 William Dufty. "Sugar Blues." Chilton Book Company, PA. Pub. 1975.

42 Splenda® is a registered trademark of McNeil Nutritionals, LLC. Available: www.splenda.com

43 Holistic Healing Web Page. "Sucralose Toxicity Information Center." Online. Accessed 9 Nov 2007. Available: www.holisticmed.com/splenda

44 Equal® and Nutrasweet® are registered trademarks of respectively the Merisant Co. and J.W. Childs Assoc. Available: www.equal.com and http://www.nutrasweet.com

45 Food and Drug Administration. "The Bressler Report." Online. Accessed 8 Aug 2007. Available as Text doc: www.dorway.com/bressler.txt

46 Dr. Betty Martini. "The Aspartame Scandal." Online. Accessed 8 Aug 2007. Available: www.ppnf.org/catalog/ppnf/Articles/Aspartame.htm

47 Michael F. Jacobson, Ph.D. "Liquid Candy–How Soft Drinks are Harming Americans' Health."

48 U. S. Department of Health and Human Services. "2005 National Survey on Drug Use & Health: National Results." Online. Accessed 9 Aug 2007. Available: www.oas.samhsa.gov/NSDUH/2k5NSDUH/2k5results.htm#Ch3

49 Ibid.

50 Ibid.

51 Ibid.

52 Abbey, A., Zawacki, T., Buck, P., Clinton, A. and P. McAuslan. "Alcohol and Sexual Assault." <u>Alcohol Research & Health</u>. Pub. Aug 2001. Vol. 25, Issue 1. (43-51). Online. Accessed 9 Aug 2007. Available as PDF: www.pubs.niaaa.nih.gov/publications/arh25-1/43-51.pdf

53 American Medical Association. "Adults Most Common Source Of Alcohol for Teens, According to Poll of Teens 13-18." Pub. 8 Aug 2005. Online. Accessed 9 Aug 2007. Available as PDF: www.harrisinteractive.com/news/newsletters/clientnews/AMA_2005_teens_alcohol.pdf

54 National Highway Traffic Safety Administration. "Traffic Safety Facts - Young Drivers." Pub. 2005. Online. Accessed 9 Aug 2007. Available as PDF: www.nrd.nhtsa.dot.gov/pdf/nrd-30/NCSA/TSF2005/2005TSF/810_630/images/810630.pdf

55 Ibid.

56 Charles de Coti-Marsh. Pp 19.

57 Shannon, S. "An Overview - Hazards of Low Level Radioactivity." Pub. Winter 1998. Online. Accessed 9 Aug 2007. Available: www.ratical.org/radiations/HoLLR.html#p4

58 World Health Organization. "Indoor air pollution and health." Online. Accessed 10 Aug 2007. Available: www.who.int/mediacentre/factsheets/fs292/en/index.html

59 Ibid.

60 Ibid.

61 Environmental Protection Agency. "Storage and Disposal of Paint Facts." Online. Accessed 10 Aug 2007. Available: www.epa.state.oh.us/pic/facts/hhwpaint.html

62 Ibid.

63 Ibid.

64   Irishhealth.com. "Smoking Increases Colon Cancer–Study." Online. Accessed 10 Aug 2007. Available: www.irishhealth.com/index.html?level=4&id=1212

65   United Health Foundation. "Prevalence of Smoking." Pub. 2003. Online. Accessed 10 Aug 2007. Available: www.unitedhealthfoundation.org/shr2004/components/smoking.html

66   Envirochex. "About Mold." Online. Accessed 13 Aug 2007. Available: www.envirochex.com/Mold/About_Mold_Spores.htm

67   Asthma and Allergy Foundation of America. "Pet Allergies." Online. Accessed 10 Aug 2007. Available: www.aafa.org/display.cfm?id=9&sub=18&cont=236

68   Arbes Jr., S., Cohn, R., Yin, M., Muilenberg, M., Burge, H., Friedman, W. and D. Zeldin. "House Dust Mite Allergen in US Beds: Results from the First National Survey of Lead and Allergens in Housing." Journal of Allergy and Clinical Immunology. Vol. 111, Issue 2. (408-14). Pub. Feb 2003. Online. Accessed 13 Aug 2007. Available as Abstract: www.jacionline.org/article/PIIS0091674902912789/abstract

69   National Institute of Allergy and Infectious Diseases. "Airborne Allergens–Something In the Air." NIH Publication No. 03-7045 Pub. April 2003. Online. Accessed 13 Aug 2007. Available as PDF: www.niaid.nih.gov/publications/allergens/airborne_allergens.pdf

70   World Health Organization. "Indoor Air Pollutants: Exposure and Health Effects." EURO Reports and Studies. Vol. 78. Pub. 1983. Online. Accessed 13 Aug. 2007. Available for Purchase: www.who.int/bookorders/WHP/detart1.jsp?sesslan=2&codlan=1&codcol=33&codcch=78

71   Agency for Toxic Substances & Disease Registry. "CERCLA Priority List of Hazardous Substances from the Agency." Pub. 2005. Online. Accessed 14 Aug 2007. Available: www.atsdr.cdc.gov/cercla/05list.html

72   Minnesota Department of Health. "Arsenic in Drinking Water and

Your Patients' Health." Online. Accessed 14 Aug 2007. Available as PDF: www.health.state.mn.us/divs/eh/groundwater/arsenicfct.pdf

73 Natural Resources Defense Council. "Arsenic in Drinking Water." Online. Accessed 14 Aug 2007. Available: www.nrdc.org/water/drinking/qarsenic.asp

74 Environmental Protection Agency. "Arsenic in Drinking Water." Online. Accessed 14 Aug 2007. Available: www.epa.gov/safewater/arsenic/basicinformation.html

75 Ibid.

76 Yiamouyiannis, J. "Water Fluoridation & Tooth Decay: Results from the 1986-1987 National Survey of US Schoolchildren." Fluoride: Journal of the International Society for Fluoride Research. Pub. April 1990. Vol. 23, Issue 2. (55-67). Online. Accessed 14 Aug 2007. Available: www.fluoridealert.org/health/teeth/caries/nidr-dmft.html

77 Physical & Theoretical Chemistry Lab. "Safety Data for Sodium fluoride." Online. Accessed 14 Aug 2007. Available: www.ptcl.chem.ox.ac.uk/MSDS/SO/sodium_fluoride.html

78 Nursery® is a registered trademark of DS Waters of America, Inc.

79 Ibid.

80 Ibid.

81 Dunnick, J. and R. Melnick. "Assessment of the Carcinogenic Potential of Chlorinated Water: Experimental Studies of Chlorine, Chloramine, and Trihalomethanes." Journal of the National Cancer Institute. Pub. 19 May 1993. Vol. 85, Issue 10. (817-22). Online. Accessed 14 Aug 2007. Available for Purchase: www.jnci.oxfordjournals.org/cgi/reprint/jnci;85/10/817

82 Kanarek, M. S. and T. B. Young. "Drinking water treatment and risk of cancer death in Wisconsin." Environmental Health Perspectives. Vol. 46. (179-86). Pub. 1982. Online. Accessed 14 Aug 2007. Avail-

able as PDF: www.ehponline.org/members/1982/046/46023.PDF

83   Morris, R., Audet, A., Angelillo, I., Chalmers, T. and F. Mosteller. "Chlorination, Chlorination By-products, and Cancer: A Meta-analysis." <u>American Journal of Public Health</u>. Pub. July 1992. Vol. 82, Issue 7. Online. Accessed 14 Aug 2007. Available as PDF: www.ajph.org/cgi/reprint/82/7/955

84   Natural Resources Defense Council. "Bottled Water-Pure Drink or Pure Hype?" Online Document. Accessed 14 Aug 2007. Available: www.nrdc.org/water/drinking/nbw.asp

85   Ibid.

86   Phillips, D., Jarvinen, J. and R. Phillips. "A Spike in Fatal Medication Errors at the Beginning of Each Month." Pharmacotherapy. Vol. 25, Issue 1. (1-9). Pub. 2005. Online. Accessed 15 Aug 2007. Available for Purchase: www.articleworks.cadmus.com/buy?c=989806&p=429278&buyopt=2&q=1

87   Jayawardena, S. et al. "Prescription Errors and the Impact of Computerized Prescription Order Entry System in a Community-based Hospital." <u>American Journal of Therapeutics</u>. Vol. 14, Issue 4. (336-40). Pub. July/Aug 2007. Online. Accessed 15 Aug 2007. Available for Purchase: www.americantherapeutics.com/pt/re/ajt/abstract.00045391-200707000-00005.htm

88   Null, G., Dean, C., Feldman, M., Rasio, D. and D. Smith. "Death by Medicine." <u>LE Magazine</u>. Pub. Aug. 2006. Available: www.lef.org/magazine/mag2006/aug2006_report_death_01.htm

89   Ibid.

90   Department of Health and Human Services. "Deaths: Preliminary Data for 2001." National Vital Statistics Report. Vol. 51, Issue 5. Pub. 14 Mar 2003. Online. Accessed 15 Aug 2007. Available as PDF: www.cdc.gov/nchs/data/nvsr/nvsr51/nvsr51_05.pdf

91   First Research Inc. "Pharmaceutical Manufacture and Sale." Pub.

May 2007. Online. Accessed 15 Aug 2007. Available: www.marketresearch.com/product/display.asp?productid=1512814&xs=r&SID=30224201-391998529-378553096

92 Null, G. et al. "Death by Medicine."

93 Pharmaceutical Research and Manufacturers of America. "Pharmaceutical Industry Profile 2006." Pub. March 2006. Online. Accessed 15 Aug 2007. Available as PDF: www.phrma.org/files/2006%20Industry%20Profile.pdf

94 National Institute for Occupational Safety and Health. "Stress ... At Work." NIOSH Publication No. 99-101. Online. Accessed 16 Aug 2007. Available: www.cdc.gov/niosh/stresswk.html

95 Ibid.

96 Ibid.

97 Ibid.

98 Centers for Disease Control and Prevention. "Healthy People 2010: Objectives for Improving Health." Online. Accessed 16 Aug 2007. Available as PDF: www.healthypeople.gov/document/pdf/Volume2/20OccSH.pdf

99 Harris Interactive. "Attitudes in the American Workplace VII - The Seventh Annual Labor Day Survey." Gallup Poll for The Marlin Company. Conducted May to June 2001. Online. Accessed 16 Aug 2007. Available as PDF: www.stress.org/2001Harris.pdf

100 The American Institute of Stress. "Job Stress." Online. Accessed 16 Aug 2007. Available: www.stress.org/job.htm

101 Ibid.

102 Frezza, E., Wachtel, M. and M. Chiriva-Internati. "The Influence of Obesity on the Risk of Developing Colon Cancer." Gut. Vol. 1. Pub. 13 Sept 2005. Online. Accessed 16 2007. Available for Purchase: www.gut.bmj.com/cgi/rapidpdf/gut.2005.073163v1.pdf

103 U.S. Census Bureau (data source). "World Life Expectancy Chart." About.com: Geography. Online. Accessed 17 Aug 2007. Available: www.geography.about.com/library/weekly/aa042000b.htm

104 Agency for Toxic Substances & Disease Registry. "CERCLA Priority List of Hazardous Substances from the Agency." Pub. 2005. Online. Accessed 14 Aug 2007. Available: www.atsdr.cdc.gov/cercla/05list.html

105 Centers for Disease Control and Prevention. "Blood and Hair Mercury Levels in Young Children and Women of Childbearing Age - United States, 1999." Morbidity and Mortality Weekly Report. Vol. 50, Issue 8. (140-3). Pub. 2 March 2001. Online. Accessed 17 Aug 2007. Available: www.cdc.gov/mmwr/preview/mmwrhtml/mm5008a2.htm

106 Luckhurst, B., Prince, E., Llopiz, J., Snodgrass, D., and E. Brothers. "Evidence of Blue Marlin (Makaira Nigricans) Spawning In Bermuda Waters and Elevated Mercury Levels in Large Specimens." Bulletin Of Marine Science. Vol. 79, Issue 3. (691–704). Pub. 2006. Online. Accessed 17 Aug 2007. Available as PDF: www.sefsc.noaa.gov/PDFdocs/Luckhurst.et.al.Bull.Mar.Sci.2006.BUM.pdf

107 Agency for Toxic Substances & Disease Registry. "CERCLA Priority List of Hazardous Substances from the Agency."

108 Zhao, Z., Hyun, J., Satsu, H., Kakuta, S. and M. Shimizu. "Oral exposure to cadmium chloride triggers an acute inflammatory response in the intestines of mice, initiated by the over-expression of tissue macrophage inflammatory protein-2 mRNA." Toxicology Letters. Vol. 164, Issue 2. (144-54). Pub. July 2006. Online. Accessed 9 Nov 2007. Available for Purchase: www.sciencedirect.com/science/journal/03784274

109 Gofman, J. "There is no safe threshold." Synapse. Vol. 38, Issue 16. Pub. 20 Jan 1994. Online. Accessed 20 Aug 2007. Available: www.ratical.org/radiation/CNR/synapse.html#quote1

110 Regan, K. "New Study Revives Old Debate About Cell Phones and Brain Tumors." TechNewsWorld. Pub. 31 March 2006. Online. Accessed 20 Aug 2007. Available: www.technewsworld.com/story/49703.html

111 Hyland, G. "Potential Adverse Health Impacts of Mobile Telephony." Pub. Dec. 1999. Online. Accessed 20 Aug 2007. Available: www.emfguru.org/EMF/hyland/hyland.htm

112 National Council on Radiation Protection & Measurements. "Biological Effects of Modulated Radiofrequency Fields." Online. Accessed 20 Aug 2007. Available for Purchase: www.ncrppublications.org/index.cfm?fm=Product.AddToCart&pid=4191384437

113 Society of Occupational Medicine. "Thyroiditis and Inflammatory Bowel Disease Associated with 50 Hz Magnetic Field Exposure." Occupational Medicine. Vol. 54, Issue 6. Pub. 2004. Online. Accessed 20 Aug 2007. Available as PDF: www.occmed.oxfordjournals.org/cgi/reprint/54/6/435

114 Weinstein, H. "Consumers win class-action status for cell phone trial." *Los Angeles Times*. Pub. 18 Aug 2007. Online. Accessed 20 Aug 2007. Available: www.heraldextra.com/content/view/234486/3. Cingular™ is a registered trademark of AT&T Knowledge Ventures.

115 United States Congress (1'st Session). "Wireless Communications and Public Safety Act of 1999." Online. Accessed 20 Aug 2007. Available: www.nena.org/govtaffairs/Leg/WICAPS99.pdf

116 Ibid.

117 Wiskemann, A., Sturml, E. and N. Klehr. "Fluorescent lighting enhances chemically induced papilloma formation and increases susceptibility to tumor challenge in mice." Journal of Cancer Research and Clinical Oncology. Vol. 112, Issue 2. (141-3). Pub. Oct 1986. Online. Accessed 21 Aug 2007. Available: www.springerlink.com/content/r38t8704u77143w5

118 Dulwich Health. "Geopathic Stress." Page 2. Online. Accessed 21

Aug 2007. Available: www.dulwichhealth.co.uk/gs2.htm

119 Amin, O. M. "Seasonal prevalence of intestinal parasites in the United States during 2000." <u>The American Journal of Tropical Medicine and Hygiene</u>. Vol. 66, Issue 6. (799-803). Pub. Jun 2002. Online. Accessed 22 Aug 2007. Available as PDF: www.ajtmh.org/cgi/reprint/66/6/799

120 Gardner, T. and D. Hill. "Treatment of Giardiasis." <u>Clinical Microbiology Reviews</u>. Vol. 14, Issue 1. (114-28). Pub. Jan 2001. Online. Accessed 23 Aug 2007. Available as PDF: www.pubmedcentral.nih.gov/picrender.fcgi?artid=88965&blobtype=pdf

121 Reves, R. et al. "Child Day Care Increases the Risk of Clinic Visits for Acute Diarrhea and Diarrhea Due to Rotavirus." <u>American Journal of Epidemiology</u>. Vol. 137, Issue 1. (97-107). Online. Accessed 23 Aug 2007. Available: www.aje.oxfordjournals.org/cgi/content/abstract/137/1/97

122 Jones, J. Kruszon-Moran, D. and M. Wilson. "Toxoplasma Gondii Infection in the United States, 1999–2000." <u>Emerging Infectious Diseases</u>. Pub. Nov. 2003. Online. Accessed 23 Aug 2007. Available: www.cdc.gov/ncidod/EID/vol9no11/03-0098.htm

123 Basavaraju, S. and P. Hotez. "Acute GI and Surgical Complications of Ascaris lumbricoides Infection." <u>Infections in Medicine</u>. Vol. 20, Issue 3. (154-9). Pub. 2003. Online. Accessed 23 Aug 2007. Available: www.medscape.com/viewarticle/451597

124 Center for Disease Control. "Parasites and Health – Enterobius." Online. Accessed 23 Aug 2007. Available: www.dpd.cdc.gov/dpdx/HTML/Enterobiasis.htm

125 Howard, K. "Walkerton96." University of Toronto Publication (date unknown). Online. Accessed 24 Aug 2007. Available as PDF: www.utsc.utoronto.ca/~gwater/index_files/Walkerton96.pdf

126 Redelings, M., Sorvillo, F. and L. Mascola. "Increase in Clostridium difficile–Related Mortality Rates, United States, 1999–2004." <u>Emerg-</u>

ing Infectious Diseases. Pub. Sept 2007. Online. Accessed 24 Aug 2007. Available as PDF: www.cdc.gov/eid/content/13/9/1417.htm

127 Ibid.

128 Centers for Disease Control and Prevention. "Division of Bacterial and Mycotic Diseases – Salmonellosis." Pub. 13 Oct. 2005. Online. Accessed 24 Aug 2007. Available: www.cdc.gov/ncidod/dbmd/diseaseinfo/salmonellosis_t.htm

129 Qing-Yi, Lu, et al. "Inhibition of prostate cancer cell growth by an avocado extract: role of lipid-soluble bioactive substances."

Subscribe to
Global Healing Center's
Free Newsletter
"Natural Health and Organic Living"

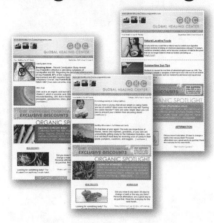

Order Dr. Group's
The Secret to Health DVD
at 50% Off!

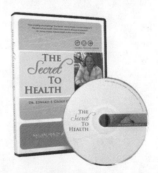

http://www.ghchealth.com/the-secret-to-health.html

Use Coupon Code: 50offdvd to receive your discount